MCQs in Medicine

MCQs in Medicine

Debra King MB, MRCP (UK),
Consultant in Geriatric Medicine,
Wirral Hospital NHS Trust

Susan J. Benbow MB, MRCP (UK),
Clinical Research Fellow,
Department of Medicine,
University of Liverpool.

With a Foreword by

Michael Lye MD, FRCP

A member of the Hodder Headline Group
LONDON • SYDNEY • AUCKLAND
Copublished in the USA by Oxford University Press, Inc., New York

First published in Great Britain in 1994
Reprinted in 1998 by Arnold,
a member of the Hodder Headline Group
338 Euston Road, London NW1 3BH

http://www.arnoldpublishers.com

Co-published in the United States of America by
Oxford University Press Inc.,
198 Madison Avenue, New York NY10016
Oxford is a registered trademark of Oxford University Press

British Library Cataloguing in Publication Data
A catalogue record for this book is available from the British Library

Library of Congress Cataloging-in-Publication Data
A catalog record for this book is available from the Library of Congress

ISBN 0-412-45710 5

Typeset in 9.5/11pt Times by Mews Photosetting
Printed and bound in Great Britain by J. W. Arrowsmith Ltd, Bristol

What do you think about this book? Or any other Arnold title?
Please send your comments to feedback.arnold@hodder.co.uk

Contents

Foreword

Academic geriatricians are always looking for an improved objective, quantifiable measure of biological ageing in humans to replace that unphysiological and arbitrary scale 'years survived'. The MCQ may be the nearest we have come yet to achieving this Holy Grail. An individual's facility with the setting and answering of MCQs separates the medical generations more surely than years. I am only grateful I was educated in a less rigorous but perhaps more 'gentlemanly' era. If one appeared before an examiner neatly dressed with clean finger nails and the examination scripts were literate essays written in fountain pen then you were in – or so it seemed. For the past 20 years we have been evolving towards much more objective and rigorous assessment of knowledge and understanding of medicine of both undergraduate and postgraduate students. This process has been exemplified by the evolution of what is now the seemingly ubiquitous MCQ.

When initially presented as objective and quantifiable measures of clinical knowledge MCQs were the subject of scorn – how could they assess the art of medicine – the grey areas of clinical decision making? However they very rapidly overcame this antediluvian scepticism and I believe they have had an effect well beyond the limited area of competence measurement. They have induced or at the very least contributed to a shift towards a more rigorous, dare one say more scientific, approach to clinical medicine. Combined with developing technology, especially in physiological measurement, this process has shifted the emphasis away from the art of medicine towards the science of medicine. In general this process has been no bad thing and has produced spectacular advances in clinical medicine and surgery. In some specialty areas however the pendulum has swung too far and there is a danger of the science overwhelming the art with a consequent decline in the humanitarian approach. If we listen, hopefully our patients will always remind us as to the best balance.

Another remarkable development over the past few years has been the decline of the generalist in medicine. Nowhere has this been more apparent than in clinical internal medicine: the general physician is now a rare and indeed endangered species. The two remaining medical generalists cover only the extremes of life. The paediatrician and the geriatrician are the proud inheritors of the generalist mantle. It is therefore entirely appropriate that this wide-ranging book has been produced by two young (? paediatric) geriatricians. The subject matter covered is enormous. The specialists may sail happily through questions in their own area of expertise but if they are like this poor individual, will find vast areas of ignorance to explore. While primarily aimed at undergraduate students, postgraduate students of any age and any seniority would benefit by 'working out' on sections within this book. After all, exercise is good for the mind as well as the body. This book represents an excellent gymnasium in the truly German meaning of the word.

Michael Lye, MD, FRCP,
Professor of Geriatric Medicine,
University of Liverpool.

Acknowledgements

We thank the following specialists for their critical review of the chapters. Their contribution has undoubtedly improved the quality of this book. However, any remaining errors whether factual or grammatical are solely our responsibility. We are also grateful to Miss Suzanne Robinson for her support and expert typing of the manuscript.

Dr S. Allard
Senior Registrar (*Haematology*)
St. George's Hospital
London

Dr A.G. Arnold
Consultant Physician (*Respiratory Medicine*)
Castle Hill Hospital and Hull Royal Infirmary
North Humberside

Professor D. Chadwick
Professor of Neurology (*Neurology*)
Walton Hospital
Liverpool

Dr G. Gill
Consultant Physician (*Endocrinology and Metabolic Disorders*)
Walton Hospital
Liverpool

Dr I. Gilmore
Consultant Physician (*Gastroenterology*)
Royal Liverpool University Hospital
Liverpool

Dr A. Harvey
Senior Lecturer in Rheumatology and Rehabilitation (*Rheumatology*)
St. James' University Hospital
Leeds

Professor M. Lye
Professor of Geriatric Medicine
University of Liverpool
Liverpool

Dr B.S. Nanda
Consultant Physician (*Infectious Disease*)
Castle Hill Hospital
North Humberside

Dr D. Pryce
Senior Registrar (*Dermatology*)
Royal Liverpool University Hospital
Liverpool

Dr J.H. Silas
Consultant Physician (*Cardiovascular Medicine*)
Wirral National Health Service Trust Hospital
Merseyside

Dr M. Yaqoob
Senior Registrar (*Renal Medcicine*)
Royal Liverpool University Hospital
Liverpool

Introduction

Multiple choice questions are an integral part of the examination of students at all stages of medical school. Likewise, they are widely used in postgraduate examinations. From the point of view of the examiner, MCQs have several attractive features: objectivity of scoring, ease of scoring (by computer) and simplicity of test interpretation. However, from the point of view of the examinee, MCQs are often a stern test of factual knowledge.

The aim of this book is to give sample questions on 10 different areas of medicine. There is, of course, no substitute for having a wide background knowledge of the topics under test. However, the following section may give some hints on how to tackle the questions.

Examination technique
The first thing to ensure is that you know the format of the questions being set. The commonest form, as in this book, is to give an introductory sentence (or stem) followed by five separate options. Each of the options in conjunction with the stem can be true or false. Other formats include only one of the five options being correct or the 'pairing' of statements from two lists. In the multiple true–false format, which is by far the most commonly used, certain grammatical clues may enable discrimination between true and false response items. For example, statements that something was 'always' or 'never' the case are usually false and statements of a less definite nature ('may be', 'usually') are more likely to be true. Although examiners should avoid setting questions with 'double' negatives they do sometimes appear. In this situation make sure that you read even more carefully than normal the stem and each option.

Before the examination starts check on the amount of time allowed and calculate the period available for each question. Throughout the examination ensure that you are keeping within your time limit. Leave some time for checking your answers or filling in any gaps. Read the stem and option carefully and make your decision.

There will always be questions where you are unsure of the answer. In these circumstances do not give up too quickly. Try and work out the answer using your knowledge. If you are still only 50% sure, then mark don't know. This is particularly important in examinations where negative marking occurs, i.e. you score -1 for a wrong answer. Remember not to spend too long over one particular stem and option. In an average examination of 60 questions, each with five options, it would be worth one-third mark.

A potentially high mark in such an examination can be lost if you fill in your answer sheet incorrectly. As you go through the paper ensure that your answers are clear and that you are placing the answer in the appropriate box or space on the answer sheet.

A good knowledge of the subject under test and familiarity with MCQ formats and grammatical clues should ensure success.

1 Cardiovascular medicine

1.1   **Regarding the jugular venous pulse (JVP):**
(a)   'a' wave is pronounced in atrial fibrillation.
(b)   'a' wave is pronounced in pulmonary stenosis.
(c)   'v' wave represents atrial filling against a closed tricuspid valve.
(d)   Normal range is +5 to +10 mmHg.
(e)   Right external jugular vein is the most reliable for assessing the JVP.

1.2   **Collapsing (waterhammer) pulse is a sign of:**
(a)   Aortic regurgitation.
(b)   Mitral stenosis.
(c)   Hyperthyroidism.
(d)   Anaemia.
(e)   Tricuspid regurgitation.

1.3   **Amiodarone:**
(a)   Has a half-life of 8 h.
(b)   Causes corneal microdeposits.
(c)   May cause a slate-grey discoloration of the skin.
(d)   May interfere with thyroid function.
(e)   Is a class IV antiarrhythmic agent.

1.4   **Impotence is a recognized side-effect of:**
(a)   Atenolol.
(b)   Spironolactone.
(c)   Frusemide.
(d)   Nifedipine.
(e)   Digoxin.

1.5   **Third heart sound:**
(a)   Is normal at any age.
(b)   May occur with mitral regurgitation.
(c)   May occur with mitral stenosis.
(d)   Is due to decreased filling of the ventricle.
(e)   May occur if a ventricular septal defect is present.

1.1
(a)	FALSE	– 'a' wave is atrial systole and is absent.
(b)	TRUE	
(c)	TRUE	
(d)	FALSE	– +3 cm measured with patient at 45° from sternal angle.
(e)	FALSE	– Right internal jugular vein should be used as it does not traverse muscle.

1.2
(a)	TRUE	
(b)	FALSE	
(c)	TRUE	
(d)	TRUE	
(e)	FALSE	– Pulse character is usually normal but prominent systolic waves occur in the JVP.

1.3
(a)	FALSE	– Half-life of 20–100 days with chronic administration.
(b)	TRUE	– Common. Rarely interferes with vision and are reversible on withdrawal of treatment.
(c)	TRUE	– Also photosensitivity occurs in 10%.
(d)	TRUE	– Hyper- or hypothyroidism may occur.
(e)	FALSE	– It is a class III drug.

1.4
(a)	TRUE	
(b)	FALSE	– Gynaecomastia is a side-effect.
(c)	FALSE	– Impotence is a side-effect of thiazide not loop diuretics.
(d)	FALSE	
(e)	FALSE	

1.5
(a)	FALSE	– It is normal in children and adults up to 40 years of age.
(b)	TRUE	– It is produced by increased ventricular filling.
(c)	FALSE	
(d)	FALSE	
(e)	TRUE	– See (b).

1.6 **Maternal rubella in the first trimester of pregnancy may cause the following in the fetus:**
(a) Fallot's tetralogy.
(b) Atrial septal defect.
(c) Aortic stenosis.
(d) Patent ductus arteriosus (PDA).
(e) Coarctation of the aorta.

1.7 **A ventricular septal defect (VSD):**
(a) Is associated with Down's syndrome.
(b) May result in Eisenmenger's syndrome.
(c) Usually closes spontaneously if large.
(d) May produce a diastolic murmur.
(e) Predisposes to infective endocarditis.

1.8 **Regarding an atrial septal defect (ASD):**
(a) An ostium primum ASD is the commonest type.
(b) An ostium secundum ASD is associated with a high incidence of infective endocarditis.
(c) Left bundle branch block is common.
(d) It produces a systolic murmur due to increased pulmonary flow.
(e) Chest X-ray shows pulmonary plethora.

1.9 **Eisenmenger's syndrome:**
(a) Is due to a left to right shunt.
(b) Results in central cyanosis.
(c) Induces polycythaemia.
(d) Is an indication for cardiac surgery.
(e) Is associated with coarctation of the aorta.

1.10 **Coarctation of the aorta:**
(a) Is usually distal to the origin of the left subclavian artery.
(b) May produce a small volume femoral pulse.
(c) Is commonly associated with a bicuspid aortic valve.
(d) Results in hypotension.
(e) Results in a double aortic knuckle on chest X-ray.

1.6
(a)	TRUE	
(b)	TRUE	– Ventricular septal defects may also occur.
(c)	FALSE	– Right-sided outflow obstruction; pulmonary valve, artery or branch stenosis.
(d)	TRUE	
(e)	FALSE	– 50% of fetuses are affected if infected in the first trimester. The systemic syndrome also includes cataracts, deafness and mental retardation.

1.7
(a)	TRUE	– Atrial septal defects are less common.
(b)	TRUE	– Right to left shunting due to pulmonary hypertension.
(c)	FALSE	– 50% of small defects close spontaneously in the first year.
(d)	TRUE	– If large, a mitral diastolic flow murmur occurs as well as the pansystolic murmur of the VSD.
(e)	TRUE	

1.8
(a)	FALSE	– Ostium secundum ASDs account for 70%.
(b)	FALSE	– Low incidence. Primum ASDs predispose to endocarditis and are usually associated with atrioventricular valve abnormalities.
(c)	FALSE	– Right bundle branch block occurs.
(d)	TRUE	– Flow through the ASD itself does not produce the murmur.
(e)	TRUE	

1.9
(a)	FALSE	– It is due to a right to left, i.e. reversal of a left to right shunt, e.g. VSD, ASD, PDA.
(b)	TRUE	
(c)	TRUE	– Due to hypoxaemia.
(d)	FALSE	– Lesion must be corrected before this serious condition develops.
(e)	FALSE	

1.10
(a)	TRUE	– In 98% of cases.
(b)	TRUE	
(c)	TRUE	– In 70% of cases and may produce an aortic systolic murmur.
(d)	FALSE	– It is a cause of hypertension in the young.
(e)	TRUE	– Due to stenosis and poststenotic dilatation.

1.11 Regarding Fallot's tetralogy:
(a) There is a VSD.
(b) Epilepsy is commoner than in the general population.
(c) Cerebral abscesses are a complication.
(d) The infant is cyanosed from birth.
(e) The chest X-ray shows pulmonary plethora.

1.12 A patent ductus arteriosus (PDA):
(a) Produces a diastolic murmur only.
(b) Is commoner in females.
(c) Usually presents with left ventricular failure.
(d) May be associated with left ventricular hypertrophy.
(e) May close if indomethacin is given in the neonatal period.

1.13 Digoxin:
(a) Toxicity may result in visual disturbances.
(b) Clearance is by the liver.
(c) Sensitivity increases in hypothyroidism.
(d) Increases conduction of the AV node and bundle of His.
(e) May cause atrial tachycardia in overdosage.

1.14 Mitral stenosis:
(a) Is commoner in men.
(b) Produces an Austin Flint murmur.
(c) May result in dysphagia.
(d) May be complicated by haemoptysis.
(e) Is associated with a collapsing pulse.

1.15 The following may be associated with aortic regurgitation:
(a) Marfan's syndrome.
(b) Right ventricular hypertrophy.
(c) Small volume pulse.
(d) Ankylosing spondylitis.
(e) Traube's sign.

1.11
(a)	TRUE	– VSD, pulmonary stenosis, over-riding of the aorta and right ventricular hypertrophy.
(b)	TRUE	
(c)	TRUE	– Due to absence of lung filter with right to left shunt (10% of cases).
(d)	FALSE	– Cyanosis appears at 3–6 months and may be precipitated by 'stress', crying or feeding.
(e)	FALSE	– Lung fields are oligaemic and pulmonary arteries small.

1.12
(a)	FALSE	– It produces a machinery murmur throughout the cardiac cycle, louder in systole.
(b)	TRUE	
(c)	FALSE	– Usually patient is asymptomatic and it is diagnosed postnatally or at a school medical.
(d)	TRUE	
(e)	TRUE	– If this is unsuccessful surgical ligation (1–5 years) is required.

1.13
(a)	TRUE	– Commonly xanthopsia (defective colour vision).
(b)	FALSE	– Clearance is by the kidneys.
(c)	TRUE	
(d)	FALSE	– Conduction is decreased.
(e)	TRUE	

1.14
(a)	FALSE	– Two-thirds of patients are women.
(b)	FALSE	– This is the mid diastolic murmur due to severe aortic regurgitation with the regurgitant jet interfering with the opening of the anterior cusp of the mitral valve.
(c)	TRUE	– A large left atrium may compress the oesophagus.
(d)	TRUE	– Due to bronchial vein rupture or pulmonary infarction.
(e)	FALSE	– Pulse is of small volume due to reduced cardiac output.

1.15
(a)	TRUE	
(b)	FALSE	– Usually left ventricular hypertrophy due to overload.
(c)	FALSE	
(d)	TRUE	
(e)	TRUE	– Eponym given to 'pistol shot' sound heard over femoral arteries.

1.16 The following are characteristic signs of aortic stenosis:
(a) Small pulse pressure.
(b) Early diastolic murmur.
(c) Arcus senilis.
(d) Ejection click in early systole.
(e) Left ventricular dilatation.

1.17 The following are causes of mitral regurgitation:
(a) Myocardial infarction.
(b) Bacterial endocarditis.
(c) Chronic obstructive pulmonary disease.
(d) Pseudoxanthoma elasticum.
(e) Acute viral pericarditis.

1.18 Regarding tricuspid regurgitation:
(a) There is a systolic murmur which increases in intensity on inspiration.
(b) Jaundice may be present.
(c) It is never due to endocarditis.
(d) The murmur is heard loudest at the apex.
(e) There is a right ventricular heave.

1.19 The following are recognized side-effects of beta-adrenoceptor antagonists:
(a) Asthma.
(b) Flushing.
(c) Nightmares.
(d) Congestive heart failure.
(e) Tachyarrhythmias.

1.20 Verapamil:
(a) Is a class IV antiarrythmic drug.
(b) Is a calcium antagonist.
(c) Usually causes diarrhoea.
(d) Causes a tachycardia.
(e) Is used in the treatment of heart failure.

1.16
(a) TRUE
(b) FALSE – Systolic ejection murmur.
(c) FALSE
(d) TRUE – This is the aortic valve opening under pressure.
(e) FALSE – Left ventricle is usually hypertrophied not dilated.

1.17
(a) TRUE – Due to papillary muscle dysfunction.
(b) TRUE – Either on a previously abnormal valve or spread from an infected aortic valve.
(c) FALSE
(d) TRUE – This is a disorder of connective tissue and results in a floppy mitral valve.
(e) FALSE

1.18
(a) TRUE – Due to increased right-sided filling (Carvallo's sign).
(b) TRUE
(c) FALSE – Increasingly seen in drug addicts.
(d) FALSE – Loudest to left of sternum in fourth intercostal space.
(e) TRUE – Due to right ventricular hypertrophy.

1.19
(a) TRUE – Due to beta-2-adrenoceptor blockade.
(b) FALSE – Causes cold hands and feet.
(c) TRUE
(d) TRUE
(e) FALSE – May cause heart block.

1.20
(a) TRUE
(b) TRUE
(c) FALSE – Commonly causes constipation.
(d) FALSE
(e) FALSE – It is negatively inotropic and may precipitate heart failure.

1.21 **The following are characteristic ECG changes with recurrent pulmonary emboli:**
(a) Right bundle branch block.
(b) Left bundle branch block.
(c) Left axis deviation.
(d) Inverted T waves in V5 and V6.
(e) Tall R waves in V1.

1.22 **Causes of left bundle branch block are:**
(a) Hypertension.
(b) Myocardial ischaemia.
(c) Atrial septal defect.
(d) Pulmonary fibrosis.
(e) Aortic stenosis.

1.23 **The following are ECG features of hypokalaemia:**
(a) μ waves.
(b) Depressed ST segments.
(c) Flat T waves.
(d) Short PR interval.
(e) Peaked T waves.

1.24 **The following may cause a sinus bradycardia:**
(a) Myxoedema.
(b) Salbutamol.
(c) Atenolol.
(d) Jaundice.
(e) Raised intracranial pressure.

1.25 **Systemic hypertension:**
(a) Increases the risk of stroke.
(b) Is usually secondary to another disease.
(c) May result in papilloedema.
(d) May be a feature of carcinoid syndrome.
(e) May be a feature of acromegaly.

1.21
(a)   TRUE
(b)   FALSE
(c)   FALSE   –   Right axis deviation due to right ventricular 'strain'.
(d)   FALSE   –   Inverted T waves in right ventricular leads V1–V3.
(e)   TRUE

1.22
(a)   TRUE
(b)   TRUE
(c)   FALSE   –   Causes right bundle branch block.
(d)   FALSE
(e)   TRUE

1.23
(a)   TRUE
(b)   TRUE
(c)   TRUE
(d)   FALSE   –   PR interval (0.12–0.2 s) lengthens.
(e)   FALSE   –   Peak T waves occur in hyperkalaemia.

1.24
(a)   TRUE
(b)   FALSE   –   Causes a tachycardia.
(c)   TRUE
(d)   TRUE
(e)   TRUE

1.25
(a)   TRUE
(b)   FALSE   –   90% of cases are primary (essential) hypertension.
(c)   TRUE   –   Grade IV hypertensive retinopathy.
(d)   FALSE
(e)   TRUE   –   Occurs in 15% of cases of acromegaly.

1.26 **The following are complications of systemic hypertension:**
(a) Right ventricular hypertrophy.
(b) Left ventricular failure.
(c) Liver function impairment.
(d) Myocardial infarction.
(e) Renal failure.

1.27 **The following are features of acute rheumatic fever:**
(a) Evidence of a staphylococcal infection.
(b) Choreiform movements.
(c) Erythema nodosum.
(d) Carey–Coombs murmur.
(e) Retinitis.

1.28 **Atrial naturetic peptide:**
(a) Is secreted from the atria in response to stretching.
(b) Decreases renal blood flow.
(c) Decreases excretion of sodium.
(d) Reduces secretion of aldosterone.
(e) Levels are increased in congestive heart failure.

1.29 **Congestive heart failure:**
(a) May result in undernutrition.
(b) Is associated with a good prognosis when treated.
(c) Is more common in the fourth decade than the sixth.
(d) May produce pulsus paradoxus.
(e) May be precipitated by enalapril.

1.30 **The following may cause ST segment depression on the ECG:**
(a) Digoxin.
(b) Angina.
(c) Left ventricular hypertrophy.
(d) Left ventricular aneurysm.
(e) Acute pericarditis.

1.26
(a)   FALSE – Left ventricular hypertrophy.
(b)   TRUE
(c)   FALSE
(d)   TRUE
(e)   TRUE

1.27
(a)   FALSE – Streptococcal infection (group A, B– haemolytic).
(b)   TRUE   – Usually in children.
(c)   TRUE   – Erythema marginatum is pathognomonic.
(d)   TRUE   – Mitral diastolic murmur due to endocarditis. This is the
                  most common murmur.
(e)   FALSE

1.28
(a)   TRUE
(b)   FALSE – It increases renal blood flow and has diuretic properties.
(c)   FALSE
(d)   TRUE
(e)   TRUE

1.29
(a)   TRUE   – Cardiac cachexia. Aetiology is multifactorial.
(b)   FALSE – Prognosis is poor.
(c)   FALSE – It is four times more common over 60 years of age.
(d)   FALSE
(e)   FALSE – ACE inhibitors are used in its treatment and improve
                  morbidity and mortality.

1.30
(a)   TRUE   – Usually concave upwards (inverted tick).
(b)   TRUE   – Particularly on exercise testing.
(c)   TRUE
(d)   FALSE – Causes persistent ST segment elevation.
(e)   FALSE – Causes convex downward ST elevation.

1.31 **The following are ECG changes of an acute inferior myocardial infarction:**
(a) Large dominant R wave in V1 and V2.
(b) ST elevation in V1–V3.
(c) ST depression in V1–V3
(d) ST elevation in II, III and aVF.
(e) A prominent p wave.

1.32 **The following are ECG features of left ventricular hypertrophy:**
(a) Left axis deviation.
(b) T wave inversion in V1–V3.
(c) Large R wave (>35 mm) in V1.
(d) p pulmonale.
(e) ST depression in V4 and V5.

1.33 **The following are causes of atrial fibrillation:**
(a) Thyrotoxicosis.
(b) Mitral stenosis.
(c) Cardiomyopathy.
(d) Bronchial carcinoma.
(e) Pulmonary embolism.

1.34 **A dissecting aneurysm of the thoracic aorta:**
(a) Is associated with ankylosing spondylitis.
(b) May result in a monoplegia.
(c) Is associated with Marfan's syndrome.
(d) Produces a systolic murmur.
(e) Has a good prognosis.

1.35 **A left atrial myxoma:**
(a) May produce a mid-diastolic murmur.
(b) Is commoner than a right atrial myxoma.
(c) Should be treated medically in the first instance.
(d) May be complicated by a stroke.
(e) Can metastasize to the lung.

1.31
(a)	FALSE	– This is the change of a true posterior infarct.
(b)	FALSE	– This is an acute anterior septal infarct.
(c)	TRUE	– These are known as reciprocal changes.
(d)	TRUE	
(e)	FALSE	

1.32
(a)	TRUE	
(b)	FALSE	– T wave inversion in V5 and V6.
(c)	FALSE	– Large R wave in V5 or V6.
(d)	FALSE	– This is a sign of a hypertrophied right atrium.
(e)	TRUE	

1.33
(a)	TRUE
(b)	TRUE
(c)	TRUE
(d)	TRUE
(e)	TRUE

1.34
(a)	FALSE	
(b)	TRUE	– Due to cerebral infarction.
(c)	TRUE	
(d)	FALSE	– A diastolic murmur of aortic regurgitation is usually present.
(e)	FALSE	– 50% die within 5 days and 90% within 6 months.

1.35
(a)	TRUE	– It mimics mitral stenosis but there is no opening snap and the murmur may be transient.
(b)	TRUE	– Three times more common.
(c)	FALSE	– Surgical removal should be performed as soon as possible.
(d)	TRUE	
(e)	FALSE	– Multiple tumours occur rarely and they never metastasize.

1.36 **A generalized low voltage ECG is associated with:**
(a) Asthma.
(b) Pericardial effusion.
(c) Myxoedema.
(d) Emphysema.
(e) Hypertension.

1.37 **The following are causes of acute pericarditis:**
(a) Coxsackie B virus.
(b) Renal failure.
(c) Systemic lupus erythematosus.
(d) Haemachromatosis.
(e) Acromegaly.

1.38 **The following are signs of cardiac tamponade:**
(a) Pulsus paradoxus.
(b) Hypertension.
(c) Inspiratory filling of the neck veins.
(d) Loud first heart sound.
(e) Displaced apex beat.

1.39 **The following are recognized complications of a myocardial infarction:**
(a) Aortic regurgitation.
(b) Hypertrophic cardiomyopathy.
(c) Ventricular septal defect.
(d) Femoral embolism.
(e) Atrial fibrillation.

1.40 **Dressler's syndrome:**
(a) Occurs 3 months after a myocardial infarction.
(b) Is associated with a high ESR.
(c) Is due to an autoimmune reaction to myocardial antigens.
(d) Often results in cardiac tamponade.
(e) Is treated with diuretics.

1.36
(a)	FALSE	
(b)	TRUE	– Due to increased distance of the heart from the chest wall.
(c)	TRUE	
(d)	TRUE	
(e)	FALSE	

1.37
(a)	TRUE	– After myocardial infarction this is the commonest cause.
(b)	TRUE	– Severe uraemia can cause pericarditis.
(c)	TRUE	
(d)	FALSE	– Associated with cardiomyopathy.
(e)	FALSE	– Associated with cardiomyopathy.

1.38
(a)	TRUE	– An increased pulse volume in expiration and reduced in inspiration.
(b)	FALSE	– Hypotension is the rule.
(c)	TRUE	– Kussmaul's sign.
(d)	FALSE	– Heart sounds are quiet.
(e)	FALSE	– The apex beat is unpalpable.

1.39
(a)	FALSE	– Mitral regurgitation due to papillary muscle dysfunction.
(b)	FALSE	
(c)	TRUE	
(d)	TRUE	– From a left ventricular mural thrombus.
(e)	TRUE	– Any arrhythmia can occur.

1.40
(a)	FALSE	– Usually 1–4 weeks.
(b)	TRUE	
(c)	TRUE	
(d)	FALSE	– This is rare.
(e)	FALSE	– Treatment is with non-steroidal anti-inflammatory drugs and/or steroids.

1.41 Regarding subacute bacterial endocarditis:
(a) *Staphylococcus aureus* is the commonest cause.
(b) Finger clubbing occurs early in the disease.
(c) Drug addicts more commonly develop infection of the mitral valve.
(d) Roth spots on the finger pulp are pathognomonic.
(e) Microscopic haematuria is usually present.

1.42 The following are features of congestive cardiomyopathy:
(a) Gallop rhythm.
(b) An ejection fraction of at least 60%.
(c) Dilated left ventricle.
(d) Tricuspid regurgitation.
(e) Pulmonary stenosis.

1.43 Regarding hypertrophic obstructive cardiomyopathy (HOCM):
(a) Inheritance is autosomol recessive.
(b) Sudden death may occur.
(c) The pulse is of small volume and 'jerky'.
(d) Ventricular arryhthmias are rare.
(e) The left ventricle is dilated.

1.44 Angiostensin converting enzyme (ACE) inhibitors:
(a) Cause peripheral vasoconstriction.
(b) Cause a chronic cough as a side-effect.
(c) Increase aldosterone levels.
(d) Decrease serum potassium.
(e) Are contraindicated in renal artery stenosis.

1.45 Regarding type IIa hyperlipidaemia: ?
(a) Cholestyamine should be prescribed in the first instance.
(b) Triglycerides are elevated.
(c) There is an increased risk of coronary artery disease.
(d) Corneal arcus may be present.
(e) It may occur secondary to nephrotic syndrome.

1.41
(a) FALSE – *Streptococcus viridans* (non-haemolytic is the commonest organism).
(b) FALSE – This is a late feature.
(c) FALSE – Tricuspid valve is infected in drug addicts.
(d) FALSE – Osler's nodes occur in finger pulps. Roth spots are seen on fundoscopy.
(e) TRUE – Due to a proliferative glomerulornephritis and/or focal embolic glomerulornephritis.

1.42
(a) TRUE
(b) FALSE – Ejection fraction is usually low (<40%).
(c) TRUE
(d) TRUE – Also mitral regurgitation due to a dilated heart.
(e) FALSE

1.43
(a) FALSE – Autosomal dominant. Equal sex distribution.
(b) TRUE
(c) TRUE – Due to outflow tract obstruction.
(d) FALSE – Common.
(e) FALSE – Left ventricular cavity is small.

1.44
(a) FALSE – Vasodilation due to decreased angiotensin II, a powerful vasoconstrictor.
(b) TRUE
(c) FALSE – This is decreased.
(d) FALSE – Potassium levels increase due to decreased aldosterone.
(e) TRUE

1.45
(a) FALSE – A low cholesterol diet is prescribed in the first instance.
(b) FALSE – Triglycerides normal. Hypercholesterolaemia is present.
(c) TRUE
(d) TRUE
(e) TRUE

1.46 **Following a myocardial infarction:**
(a) Driving should be discontinued for 3 months.
(b) The highest serum creatine phosphokinase occurs on day 3.
(c) Pyrexia is common after 2 days.
(d) Thrombolysis reduces mortality if given within 6 h.
(e) All patients would benefit from percutaneous transluminal coronary angioplasty.

1.47 **The management of unstable angina includes:**
(a) Aspirin.
(b) An exercise stress test.
(c) Anticoagulation.
(d) Nitrates.
(e) Digoxin.

1.48 **Indications for coronary artery bypass grafting include:**
(a) Stenosis (>80%) of the left anterior descending artery.
(b) Disease effecting the right main coronary artery only.
(c) Proximal obstruction to at least two major arteries.
(d) Syndrome X.
(e) An ejection fraction of <10%.

1.49 **Echocardiography:**
(a) Makes use of ultrasound waves.
(b) Is unable to assess left ventricular function.
(c) Is able to demonstrate a pericardial effusion.
(d) Requires a general anaesthetic.
(e) Should be performed in all cases of heart failure.

1.50 **The following are features of left ventricular failure:**
(a) Kerley B lines on the chest X-ray.
(b) Peripheral oedema.
(c) Pulsus alternans.
(d) Pulsus bisferiens.
(e) Orthopnoea.

1.46
(a)	FALSE	– Stop driving for 4 weeks.
(b)	FALSE	– Peak levels are after 24 h.
(c)	TRUE	
(d)	TRUE	
(e)	FALSE	– There are specific indications for this technique.

1.47
(a)	TRUE	– Aspirin reduces the incidence of myocardial infarction and mortality.
(b)	FALSE	– This is contraindicated.
(c)	TRUE	– Intravenous heparin.
(d)	TRUE	
(e)	FALSE	– Only if patient is in atrial fibrillation.

1.48
(a)	TRUE	
(b)	FALSE	
(c)	TRUE	
(d)	FALSE	– The coronary arteries are normal.
(e)	FALSE	– This is a contraindication due to increased operative mortality.

1.49
(a)	TRUE	
(b)	FALSE	
(c)	TRUE	
(d)	FALSE	– It is a non-invasive technique. Transoesophageal echocardiography requires a local anaesthetic.
(e)	TRUE	

1.50
(a)	TRUE	
(b)	FALSE	– Feature of right ventricular failure.
(c)	TRUE	
(d)	FALSE	– Double impulse pulse due to mixed aortic valve diseae.
(e)	TRUE	

1.51 Congestive heart failure results in:
(a) Increased serum levels of aldosterone.
(b) Peripheral vasodilatation.
(c) Decreased sympathetic nervous system activity.
(d) Increased peripheral resistance.
(e) Retention of sodium.

1.52 Fourth heart sound:
(a) Is due to ventricular filling.
(b) Occurs in pulmonary stenosis.
(c) Is pathological.
(d) Occurs in systemic hypertension.
(e) Is common in the neonate.

1.53 Splitting of the second heart sound with respiration:
(a) Is normal on inspiration.
(b) Is fixed in aortic stenosis.
(c) Is reversed in aortic stenosis.
(d) Is reversed in right bundle branch block.
(e) Is reversed in left bundle branch block.

1.54 The following are recognized associations of a left ventricular aneurysm:
(a) Persistent ST segment depression on the ECG.
(b) Supraventricular arrythmias.
(c) Left ventricular failure.
(d) Ventricular tachycardia.
(e) Stroke.

1.55 Recognized features of Wolff–Parkinson–White Syndrome (WPW) include:
(a) Widened QRS complex.
(b) j wave.
(c) Delta wave.
(d) Recurrent supraventricular tachycardia.
(e) Prolonged PR interval.

1.51
(a)   TRUE
(b)   FALSE – Vasoconstriction due to increased angiotensin II and noradrenaline.
(c)   FALSE
(d)   TRUE
(e)   TRUE

1.52
(a)   FALSE – It is due to atrial contraction.
(b)   TRUE
(c)   TRUE
(d)   TRUE
(e)   FALSE

1.53
(a)   TRUE
(b)   FALSE – It is reversed (P_2A_2 in expiration) due to delayed left ventricular ejection.
(c)   TRUE
(d)   FALSE – It is fixed (A_2P_2 in inspiration and expiration).
(e)   TRUE

1.54
(a)   FALSE – Persistent ST elevation.
(b)   FALSE
(c)   TRUE
(d)   TRUE
(e)   TRUE – Due to systemic embolus from thrombus in aneurysm which is common.

1.55
(a)   TRUE
(b)   FALSE – This occurs in hypothermia.
(c)   TRUE – A slurred upstroke on the R wave.
(d)   TRUE
(e)   FALSE – Short PR interval (0.1–0.12 s).

1.56 **The following drugs may be used to treat ventricular tachycardia:**
(a) Verapamil.
(b) Lignocaine.
(c) Amiodarone.
(d) Phenytoin.
(e) Atenolol.

1.57 **Cardiogenic shock:**
(a) Has a high mortality.
(b) Results in polyuria.
(c) May result in lactic acidosis.
(d) Results in peripheral vasoconstriction.
(e) Requires the use of specific chronotropic drugs.

1.58 **Indications for emergency surgery in infective endocarditis are:**
(a) Mitral stenosis.
(b) Intractable heart failure.
(c) Resistent infection of a valve prosthesis.
(d) Dilated cardiomyopathy.
(e) Hypertrophic obstructive cardiomyopathy.

1.59 **The following are risk factors for coronary artery disease:**
(a) Diet rich in unsaturated fats.
(b) Diabetes mellitus.
(c) Hypercholesterolaemia.
(d) Excessive exercise.
(e) Heroin addiction.

1.60 **Raynaud's phenomenon may be associated with:**
(a) Cervical rib.
(b) Obesity.
(c) Scleroderma.
(d) Oral contraceptive pill.
(e) Thyrotoxicosis.

1.56
(a)	FALSE
(b)	TRUE – This is the first drug of choice.
(c)	TRUE
(d)	TRUE
(e)	FALSE

1.57
(a)	TRUE – Mortality approximately 80%.
(b)	FALSE – Oliguria due to pre-renal failure.
(c)	TRUE – Due to hypoxia causing anaerobic metabolism.
(d)	TRUE
(e)	FALSE – Inotropes are required.

1.58
(a)	FALSE
(b)	TRUE
(c)	TRUE
(d)	FALSE
(e)	FALSE – Patients with HOCM are susceptible to endocarditis.

1.59
(a)	FALSE – Saturated fats increase risk.
(b)	TRUE
(c)	TRUE
(d)	FALSE
(e)	FALSE

1.60
(a)	TRUE
(b)	FALSE – Not directly associated with this, i.e. not a cause.
(c)	TRUE
(d)	TRUE
(e)	FALSE – This is associated with warm extremities.

2 Respiratory medicine

2.1 Finger clubbing may be associated with:
(a) Chronic bronchitis.
(b) Bronchiectasis.
(c) Pulmonary fibrosis.
(d) Bronchial carcinoma.
(e) Asthma.

2.2 Chronic bronchitis:
(a) Is a diagnosis which is usually made on chest X-ray appearances.
(b) Is commoner in men.
(c) Is more prevalent in the USA than the UK.
(d) Results in an increased FEV_1.
(e) May cause severe hypoxia during REM sleep.

2.3 Emphysema:
(a) Is a clinical diagnosis.
(b) Almost always is accompanied by right heart failure.
(c) Often results in purse-lip breathing.
(d) Causes an increased total lung capacity and reduced transfer factor.
(e) Results in copious sputum production.

2.4 Regarding pneumonia:
(a) *Streptococcus pneumoniae* is the most common aetiological organism.
(b) If occuring during an influenza epidemic then *Klebsiella pneumoniae* is the usual cause.
(c) If caused by *Legionella pneumophila* (Legionnaires' disease) it is sometimes associated with myalgia and renal failure.
(d) If caused by *Mycoplasma pneumoniae*, high-dose intravenous benzyl-penicillin should be used.
(e) If staphylococcal, lung abscesses may occur.

2.5 Miliary tuberculosis:
(a) Most commonly follows primary infection.
(b) Is classically associated with lobar consolidation.
(c) May result in pancytopenia.
(d) May cause hepatosplenomegaly.
(e) Is difficult to diagnose in the elderly because of non-specific symptoms.

2.1
(a) FALSE
(b) TRUE
(c) TRUE
(d) TRUE
(e) FALSE – May occur in all forms of suppurative lung disease, cyanotic congenital heart disease, bacterial endocarditis, cirrhosis, inflammatory bowel disease and coeliac disease.

2.2
(a) FALSE – The diagnosis is clinical: cough productive of sputum on most days for 3 months for at least 2 years.
(b) TRUE
(c) FALSE – Prevalence is higher in the UK than any other country. Also related to smoking, lower social class and atmospheric pollution.
(d) FALSE – The FEV_1/FVC is usually less than 75%.
(e) TRUE – Continuous oxygen therapy for 15 of the 24 h reduces mortality.

2.3
(a) FALSE – The diagnosis is pathological; dilatation of the terminal airways distal to the terminal bronchioles with destruction of their walls.
(b) FALSE – Heart failure is unusual.
(c) TRUE – This keeps the intrabronchial pressure above that of the surrounding alveoli and prevents collapse of the bronchial walls produced by air trapped in the surrounding alveoli.
(d) TRUE
(e) FALSE – Sputum volume is usually small.

2.4
(a) TRUE
(b) FALSE – Usually staphylococcal pneumonia.
(c) TRUE
(d) FALSE – The organism is sensitive to tetracyclines and erythromycin.
(e) TRUE

2.5
(a) FALSE
(b) FALSE – Classical chest X-ray findings in 50% are multiple 'millet seed' sized nodules throughout both lung fields.
(c) TRUE – Due to invasion of the bone marrow.
(d) TRUE
(e) TRUE – Unfortunately it is all too often diagnosed at post mortem.

2.6 **Regarding a lung abscess:**
(a) It may complicate bronchial carcinoma.
(b) It may be a sequel to *Klebsiella* pneumonia.
(c) Clubbing may develop.
(d) It usually presents incidentally as a cavity with a fluid level on a routine chest X-ray.
(e) Surgical excision is often required.

2.7 **Transfer factor (TLco) is usually increased in the following:**
(a) Emphysema.
(b) Pulmonary fibrosis.
(c) Polycythaemia rubra vera.
(d) Goodpasture's syndrome.
(e) Anaemia.

2.8 **The following may cause a pleural effusion which is an exudate : protein >30 g/1:**
(a) Pneumonia.
(b) Left ventricular failure.
(c) Pulmonary embolism.
(d) Nephrotic syndrome.
(e) Systemic lupus erythematosus.

2.9 **Regarding carcinoma of the bronchus:**
(a) It is commoner in men.
(b) Oat cell carcinoma is the commonest type.
(c) Parathyroid-like hormone may be produced by a squamous cell tumour resulting in hypercalcaemia.
(d) Oat cell carcinoma responds to chemotherapy.
(e) It may be associated with Eaton Lambert syndrome.

2.10 **A bronchial adenoma:**
(a) Is always benign.
(b) Is usually a 'carcinoid' tumour histologically.
(c) Most often is peripheral.
(d) May occur in association with rheumatoid arthritis.
(e) Often presents with haemoptysis.

2.6

(a)	TRUE		
(b)	TRUE		
(c)	TRUE		
(d)	FALSE	–	Usually the patient is very ill with a swinging fever and a chest X-ray helps to confirm the diagnosis.
(e)	FALSE	–	This is unusual. Treatment with postural drainage and antibiotics usually suffice.

2.7

(a)	FALSE	–	It is decreased.
(b)	FALSE	–	It is decreased.
(c)	TRUE		
(d)	TRUE	–	This rare disease is caused by antibody development against basement membrane in the glomeruli and lungs. It results in lung haemorrhages and renal failure.
(e)	FALSE	–	It is decreased. Transfer factor expresses the ability of the lungs to transfer carbon monoxide from the alveoli to the blood.

2.8

(a)	TRUE		
(b)	FALSE	–	May cause an effusion which is a transudate.
(c)	TRUE		
(d)	FALSE	–	May cause an effusion which is a transudate.
(e)	TRUE		

2.9

(a)	TRUE	–	Although it is becoming commoner in women because of the increase in smoking among them.
(b)	FALSE	–	Squamous cell is commonest (40%) followed by oat cell (small cell), undifferentiated (large cell) and adenocarcinoma.
(c)	TRUE		
(d)	TRUE		
(e)	TRUE		

2.10

(a)	FALSE	–	There is a risk of neoplastic change.
(b)	TRUE	–	90% are histologically carcinoid tumours.
(c)	FALSE	–	Usually occurs in major bronchi.
(d)	FALSE		
(e)	TRUE		

2.11 Pulmonary fibrosis can be present in:
(a) Paraquat poisoning.
(b) Rheumatoid arthritis.
(c) Sarcoidosis.
(d) Chronic bronchitis.
(e) Extrinsic asthma.

2.12 Regarding asthma:
(a) It is usually associated with atopy in the late-onset type.
(b) Peak Expiratory Flow Rate (PEFR) is the highest in the morning.
(c) Acute attacks respond to beta-2-adrenoceptor antagonists.
(d) Steroids should always be used in an acute attack.
(e) Surgical (subcutaneous) emphysema may occur.

2.13 Sarcoidosis:
(a) Is commoner in men.
(b) Is a common cause of erythema nodosum.
(c) May cause hypercalcaemia.
(d) Most commonly shows chest X-ray changes of diffuse fibrosis.
(e) May cause parotitis.

2.14 The following are true of pulmonary emboli:
(a) Chest X-ray may be normal.
(b) $PaCO_2$ is usually more than 6 kPa.
(c) Pulmonary angiography is most likely to give the diagnosis.
(d) It is rare in pregnancy.
(e) Atrial fibrillation may occur.

2.15 Regarding cystic fibrosis:
(a) The condition is caused by a Mendelian dominant gene.
(b) Malabsorption may occur.
(c) Tuberculosis occurs more commonly than in the general population.
(d) Salt concentration in sweat is low.
(e) *Pseudomonas aeruginosa* in the sputum is common at presentation.

2.11
(a)   TRUE
(b)   TRUE
(c)   TRUE
(d)   FALSE
(e)   FALSE

2.12
(a)   FALSE   –   Usually extrinsic asthma caused by type I hyper-
              sensitivity reaction presents in childhood.
(b)   FALSE   –   Usually low, 'morning dip' in peak flow.
(c)   FALSE   –   Beta-2-agonists, e.g. salbutamol dilate bronchial smooth
              muscle.
(d)   TRUE
(e)   TRUE   –   May occur after rupture of the alveoli causing a
              pneumomediastinum and air rising to the shoulders
              (pneumothorax may also be present).

2.13
(a)   FALSE   –   Five times more common in women.
(b)   TRUE
(c)   TRUE
(d)   FALSE   –   Commonest X-ray change is bilateral hilar enlargement
              due to lymphadenopathy.
(e)   TRUE

2.14
(a)   TRUE
(b)   FALSE   –   Usually there is hypoxia with a normal $PaCO_2$.
(c)   TRUE
(d)   FALSE
(e)   TRUE

2.15
(a)   FALSE   –   Recessive gene carried by 1 in 20 of the population.
(b)   TRUE
(c)   TRUE
(d)   FALSE   –   It is high and may lead to salt depletion in hot climates
              and during fever.
(e)   FALSE   –   Colonization by this organism usually occurs when lung
              damage is well established late in the disease.

2.16 **Regarding mesothelioma:**
(a) This may develop 20–40 years after asbestos exposure.
(b) Metastasis is very rare.
(c) It is a tumour of the alveolar cells.
(d) Chest pain is uncommon.
(e) Most patients survive 10 years after the diagnosis.

2.17 **The following pulmonary phenomena are associated with rheumatoid arthritis:**
(a) Pleural effusion.
(b) Bronchiectasis.
(c) Pulmonary fibrosis.
(d) Pulmonary emboli.
(e) Intrapulmonary nodules.

2.18 **Bronchiectasis may produce the following:**
(a) Pneumothorax.
(b) Lung abscess.
(c) Cerebral abscess.
(d) Left heart failure.
(e) Halitosis.

2.19 **The following are true:**
(a) Kerley B lines occur in chronic bronchitis.
(b) Acute asthma is associated with negligible mortality.
(c) An apical bronchial carcinoma (Pancoasts' tumour) may result in Horner's syndrome.
(d) Asbestos bodies in sputum are indicative of a mesothelioma.
(e) ECG in recurrent pulmonary emboli may show a left ventricular strain pattern.

2.20 **The following are true of left lower lobe collapse:**
(a) Trachea is deviated to the right.
(b) It may follow an attack of asthma.
(c) There are bronchial breath sounds audible.
(d) It may be due to a bronchial carcinoma.
(e) Left hemidiaphragm is usually elevated.

2.16
(a)   TRUE
(b)   TRUE
(c)   FALSE – It is a tumour of the pleura.
(d)   FALSE
(e)   FALSE – Most die within 1–2 years and treatment is palliative.

2.17
(a)   TRUE
(b)   FALSE
(c)   TRUE
(d)   FALSE
(e)   TRUE

2.18
(a)   FALSE
(b)   TRUE
(c)   TRUE
(d)   FALSE – Usually right heart failure secondary to pulmonary hypertension (cor pulmonale).
(e)   TRUE

2.19
(a)   FALSE – These are lines representing interstitial oedema in a patient with left ventricular failure.
(b)   FALSE
(c)   TRUE
(d)   FALSE – They are indicative only of previous asbestos exposure.
(e)   FALSE – Usually right ventricular strain.

2.20
(a)   FALSE – The trachea is pulled to the side of collapse.
(b)   TRUE   – Usually due to obstruction by inspissated sputum.
(c)   FALSE
(d)   TRUE
(e)   TRUE

2.21 Haemoptysis is commonly associated with:
(a) Bronchiectasis.
(b) Bronchial carcinoma.
(c) Asthma.
(d) Mitral stenosis.
(e) Pulmonary fibrosis.

2.22 Central cyanosis:
(a) Is best detected in the hands.
(b) Is present if there is an excess of 5 g/dl of reduced haemoglobin.
(c) Is apparent even in the presence of severe anaemia.
(d) Usually results in a flapping tremor.
(e) Is produced by cold weather.

2.23 The following are clinical signs of a large pleural effusion:
(a) Increased vocal fremitus.
(b) Increased vocal resonance.
(c) Dull percussion.
(d) Wheeze.
(e) Bronchial breathing.

2.24 The following are clinical signs of a right pneumothorax:
(a) Tracheal deviation to right.
(b) Right-sided bronchial breath sounds.
(c) Decreased vocal resonance on the left.
(d) Dull percussion on right.
(e) Whispering pectoriloquy on right.

2.25 The following are clinical features of hypercapnia:
(a) Central cyanosis.
(b) Papilloedema.
(c) Bounding pulse.
(d) Vomiting.
(e) Headache.

2.21
(a)	TRUE	– Due to destruction of bronchial vessels.
(b)	TRUE	– Often it is the presenting symptom.
(c)	FALSE	
(d)	TRUE	– Due to pulmonary hypertension and bronchial vessel rupture.
(e)	FALSE	

2.22
(a)	FALSE	– It is best seen in the tongue and lips.
(b)	TRUE	
(c)	FALSE	– If hypoxia is present in severe anaemia there will not be enough reduced haemoglobin to produce central cyanosis.
(d)	FALSE	– Carbon dioxide retention causes this.
(e)	FALSE	– This produces peripheral cyanosis which is always present with central cyanosis. Central cyanosis is due to disease of the heart or lungs.

2.23
(a)	FALSE	– This is decreased as is vocal resonance due to the decreased conduction of air to the chest wall.
(b)	FALSE	
(c)	TRUE	
(d)	FALSE	
(e)	TRUE	– May occur due to compression of smaller bronchi by large effusion.

2.24
(a)	FALSE	– Deviation is to opposite side especially in tension pneumothorax.
(b)	FALSE	– Breath sounds are absent.
(c)	FALSE	– Decreased on right.
(d)	FALSE	– Percussion note is hyper-resonant.
(e)	FALSE	– This is absent. When present it indicates consolidation.

2.25
(a)	FALSE	– This is a feature of hypoxia.
(b)	TRUE	– Due to vasodilatatory effect of carbon dioxide.
(c)	TRUE	– Due to vasodilatatory effect of carbon dioxide.
(d)	FALSE	
(e)	TRUE	– see (b).

2.26 **The following are causes of bronchiectasis:**
(a) Kartagener's syndrome.
(b) Whooping cough.
(c) Tuberculosis.
(d) Chronic bronchitis.
(e) Allergic bronchopulmonary aspergillosis.

2.27 **Causes of type I respiratory failure are:**
(a) Acute asthma.
(b) Muscular dystrophy.
(c) Myasthenia gravis.
(d) Left ventricular failure.
(e) Thromboembolism.

2.28 **Normal values of Peak Expiratory Flow Rate (l/min) vary with:**
(a) Sex.
(b) Race.
(c) Height.
(d) Shoe size.
(e) Hair colour.

2.29 **Pulmonary surfactant:**
(a) Increases surface tension.
(b) Is defective in respiratory distress syndrome of the new born.
(c) Is mainly found in the trachea.
(d) Activity and production is increased in pulmonary embolism.
(e) Is insoluble in water.

2.30 **The following may cause 'miliary' mottling on the chest X-ray:**
(a) Sarcoidosis.
(b) Pneumoconiosis.
(c) Lymphangitis carcinomatosis.
(d) Hydatid cysts.
(e) Hamartomas.

2.26

(a)   TRUE   –   Features are dextrocardia, situs inversus, infertility, sinusitis and otitis media. Patients have ciliary immotility.

(b)   TRUE

(c)   TRUE

(d)   FALSE

(e)   TRUE   –   Causes proximal airway bronchiectasis.

2.27

(a)   TRUE   –   Reduced PO_2 and normal or low PCO_2.

(b)   FALSE   –   Causes type II respiratory failure, hypoxaemia with hypercapnia.

(c)   FALSE   –   Causes type II respiratory failure.

(d)   TRUE

(e)   TRUE

2.28

(a)   TRUE

(b)   TRUE

(c)   TRUE

(d)   FALSE

(e)   FALSE

2.29

(a)   FALSE   –   It reduces surface tension in small cavities (alveoli) and therefore prevents them collapsing.

(b)   TRUE

(c)   FALSE   –   It is a lipoprotein mainly found at the air–fluid interface in the alveoli.

(d)   FALSE   –   Underperfusion decreases production of surfactant and may explain the collapse associated with pulmonary embolism.

(e)   TRUE

2.30

(a)   TRUE

(b)   TRUE

(c)   TRUE

(d)   FALSE   –   Usually single and produces a rounded shadow.

(e)   FALSE   –   A benign rounded tumour of lung.

2.31 Beta-2-adrenoceptor agonists:
(a) Include aminophylline.
(b) Increase cyclic AMP in bronchial smooth muscle and mast cells.
(c) Are best given orally.
(d) May produce a tremor.
(e) May cause hypokalaemia.

2.32 The following are recognized side-effects of theophylline:
(a) Hyperkalaemia.
(b) Vomiting.
(c) Convulsions.
(d) Tachyarrythmias.
(e) Sedation.

2.33 Regarding staphylococcal pneumonia:
(a) Gram-negative coccus is isolated from the sputum.
(b) It may be a common sequel to influenza.
(c) It is usually a mild illness in the young.
(d) It is treated with benzylpenicillin.
(e) It may be complicated by a cerebral abscess.

2.34 Legionnaire's disease:
(a) Is treated with intravenous cephalosporins.
(b) May be accompanied by acute renal failure.
(c) Is caused by a gram negative bacillus.
(d) Is associated with a negligible mortality.
(e) May be transmitted via air conditioning systems.

2.35 Regarding pneumocystis carinii pneumonia:
(a) Haemoptysis is a prominent symptom.
(b) Diagnosis is by sputum culture.
(c) Treatment is with high-dose cotrimoxazole.
(d) It is more common in the immunosuppressed.
(e) Chest X-ray shows lobar consolidation.

2.31
(a) FALSE – This is a xanthine derivative and is a phosphodiesterases (enzyme which breaks down cyclic AMP) inhibitor.
(b) TRUE
(c) FALSE – Inhalation is best form of delivery so the drug reaches site of action with fewer side-effects.
(d) TRUE
(e) TRUE

2.32
(a) FALSE – May cause hypokalaemia.
(b) TRUE – Therapeutic range = 10–20 mg/1 but there is a narrow margin between the therapeutic and toxic dose.
(c) TRUE
(d) TRUE
(e) FALSE – May cause insomnia.

2.33
(a) FALSE – *Staphylococcus* is Gram-positive.
(b) TRUE
(c) FALSE – It is a severe pneumonia with a significant mortality.
(d) FALSE – Treatment is with flucloxacillin 500 mg four times daily orally or intravenously. Fusidic acid if penicillin sensitive.
(e) TRUE – Remote septic systemic emboli may occur as well as lung abscesses.

2.34
(a) FALSE – Erythromycin is the drug of choice. Tetracycline may be as effective.
(b) TRUE
(c) TRUE – *Legionella pneumophila.*
(d) FALSE – High (20%).
(e) TRUE

2.35
(a) FALSE – Uncommon. Breathlessness and tachypnoea are the main features.
(b) TRUE
(c) TRUE – Or pentamidine.
(d) TRUE – e.g. patients with AIDS.
(e) FALSE – There is widespread mottling which is slowly progressive.

2.36 **Regarding antituberculous treatment:**
(a) Concomitant administration of pyridoxine with isoniazid prevents development of peripheral neuropathy in slow acetylators.
(b) Drug treatment should be continued for 18 months.
(c) Rifampicin colours the urine red.
(d) Rifampicin can reduce the effect of the oral contraceptive pill.
(e) Ethambutol may cause optic neuritis.

2.37 **The following cause bronchioconstriction:**
(a) Adrenaline.
(b) Ipratropium Bromide.
(c) Histamine.
(d) Prostaglandin F_2.
(e) Kinins.

2.38 **Asthma:**
(a) Is commoner in children.
(b) Mortality has decreased substantially in the last 50 years.
(c) Is associated with eosinophil infiltration of the bronchial wall.
(d) Mortality is greatest in the afternoon.
(e) May result in a pneumomediastinum.

2.39 **The following are features of extrinsic allergic alveolitis:**
(a) Type III hypersensitivity reaction.
(b) Persistent fine crackles on chest auscultation.
(c) Myalgia.
(d) Increased transfer factor.
(e) Fever.

2.40 **The following may be associated with bronchial carcinoma:**
(a) Erythema nodosum.
(b) Acanthosis nigricans.
(c) Proximal myopathy.
(d) Peripheral neuropathy.
(e) Erythema marginatum.

2.36
(a)	TRUE	– Metabolized by liver, includes acetylation. Slow acetylation is common in Orientals.
(b)	FALSE	– Treatment is with rifampicin, isoniazid, ethambutol and pyrazinamide for 2 months, then rifampicin and isoniazid for a further 6 months.
(c)	TRUE	
(d)	TRUE	– It induces liver enzymes and increases the breakdown of the pill.
(e)	TRUE	

2.37
(a)	FALSE	
(b)	FALSE	– This is an anticholinergic drug and it causes bronchodilatation.
(c)	TRUE	– Asthmatics are more sensitive to histamine induced bronchospasm than normals.
(d)	TRUE	
(e)	TRUE	

2.38
(a)	TRUE	
(b)	FALSE	– Mortality has remained constant for many years. 1500 deaths annually in the UK.
(c)	TRUE	
(d)	FALSE	– Deaths most common at night and in early morning. Mortality in UK is increased in the summer.
(e)	TRUE	– Due to rupture of the alveoli; leaking air into the mediastinum. Pneumothorax and subcutaneous emphysema are other complications.

2.39
(a)	TRUE	– Precipitins can be demonstrated in the serum (i.e. antibodies to certain antigens).
(b)	TRUE	
(c)	TRUE	
(d)	FALSE	– It is reduced due to thickening of the alveolar membrane.
(e)	TRUE	

2.40
(a)	FALSE	
(b)	TRUE	– Pigmented areas under the arms, breasts and in the groin. It is a skin manifestation of underlying malignancy.
(c)	TRUE	
(d)	TRUE	
(e)	FALSE	– This is pathognomonic of rheumatic fever.

2.41 **The following are characteristic of cryptogenic fibrosing alveolitis:**
(a) Onset in early teens.
(b) Cough productive of copious amounts of sputum.
(c) Obstructive ventilatory defect.
(d) Finger clubbing.
(e) Wheezes on auscultation of the chest.

2.42 **The following may be associated with sarcoidosis:**
(a) Erythema nodosum.
(b) Hypercalcaemia.
(c) Bone cysts.
(d) Progressive destructive arthopathy.
(e) Facial nerve palsy.

2.43 **The following are side-effects of long-term steroids:**
(a) Osteoporosis.
(b) Cushing's disease.
(c) Hypertension.
(d) Diabetes mellitus.
(e) Haematuria.

2.44 **Primary pulmonary hypertension:**
(a) May give rise to a Graham Steell murmur.
(b) Is commoner in women.
(c) Usually results in an absent 'a' wave in the JVP.
(d) May be treated with intravenous prostacyclin.
(e) Has a neglibible mortality.

2.45 **The following are characteristic features of cor pulmonale:**
(a) Tapping apex beat.
(b) Left axis deviation on the ECG.
(c) Hypoxaemia.
(d) Parasternal heave.
(e) Aortic valve disease.

2.41
(a)	FALSE	– Most common in late middle age.
(b)	FALSE	– Cough is unproductive. Dyspnoea is an early symptom.
(c)	FALSE	– Restrictive ventilatory defect.
(d)	TRUE	– Occurs in two thirds of cases.
(e)	FALSE	– Crackles on inspiration most marked at the end of inspiration are most characteristic.

2.42
(a)	TRUE	– Sarcoidosis is the commonest cause of this in the UK.
(b)	TRUE	– Due to increased absorption of calcium and may cause nephrocalcinosis and renal failure.
(c)	TRUE	
(d)	FALSE	– Polyarthritis is common but is not destructive.
(e)	TRUE	– Due to meningeal involvement.

2.43
(a)	TRUE	
(b)	FALSE	– This is due to an adenoma of the pituitary gland.
(c)	TRUE	
(d)	TRUE	
(e)	FALSE	

2.44
(a)	TRUE	– This is the murmur of pulmonary regurgitation (early diastolic).
(b)	TRUE	
(c)	FALSE	– Only if in atrial fibrillation. The 'a' wave is usually prominent due to atrial hypertrophy.
(d)	TRUE	– This lowers pulmonary vascular resistance.
(e)	FALSE	– It is usually fatal within 3 years.

2.45
(a)	FALSE	– This is a sign of mitral stenosis.
(b)	FALSE	– Usually right axis deviation and right ventricular 'strain' pattern.
(c)	TRUE	
(d)	TRUE	– Due to right ventricular hypertrophy.
(e)	FALSE	– Cor pulmonale is heart failure developing as a consequence of chronic respiratory disease.

2.46 **Regarding an empyema:**
(a) It is usually an incidental finding on a chest X-ray.
(b) It may follow a ruptured oesophagus.
(c) It may follow *Klebsiella* pneumonia.
(d) Aspiration is contraindicated.
(e) It becomes the seat of anaerobic infections.

2.47 **The following may be associated with surgical emphysema:**
(a) Intermittent positive pressure ventilation.
(b) Asthma.
(c) Tension pneumothorax.
(d) Ruptured oesophagus.
(e) Sarcoidosis.

2.48 **The following are characteristic of adult respiratory distress syndrome (ARDS):**
(a) It may develop during septicaemic shock.
(b) Chest X-ray shows widespread diffuse shadowing.
(c) It is accompanied by pulmonary hypertension.
(d) Surfactant is secreted in excessive amounts.
(e) Majority of victims recover.

2.49 **The following are signs of left lower lobe consolidation:**
(a) Deviation of the trachea to the right.
(b) Hyper-resonant percussion note.
(c) Increased vocal resonance.
(d) Bronchial breath sounds.
(e) Herpes labialis.

2.50 **Silicosis:**
(a) Predisposes to pulmonary oedema.
(b) Predisposes to tuberculosis.
(c) Is associated with farming.
(d) May cause a restrictive ventilatory defect.
(e) May cause a reduced transfer factor.

2.46
(a)	FALSE	–	The patient is usually ill with a swinging fever.
(b)	TRUE	–	It is usually left-sided.
(c)	TRUE		
(d)	FALSE	–	It is essential to drain the pus. This and antibiotics are the mainstay of treatment.
(e)	TRUE		

2.47
(a)	TRUE
(b)	TRUE
(c)	TRUE
(d)	TRUE
(e)	FALSE

2.48
(a)	TRUE	–	Other causes are aspiration, pulmonary embolism and trauma.
(b)	TRUE		
(c)	FALSE	–	This is normmal.
(d)	FALSE	–	There is decreased surfactant production and increased pulmonary permeability.
(e)	FALSE	–	It has a high mortality (60%).

2.49
(a)	FALSE	–	Deviation to left only if associated with collapse.
(b)	FALSE	–	Percussion is dull.
(c)	TRUE		
(d)	TRUE		
(e)	FALSE	–	This often accompanies streptococcal lobar pneumonia but is not a specific sign of left lower lobe consolidation.

2.50
(a)	FALSE		
(b)	TRUE		
(c)	FALSE	–	Due to exposure to silicaceous dust, e.g. quarrying, mining, sandblasting.
(d)	TRUE		
(e)	TRUE		

2.51 Exposure to asbestos may cause:
(a) Pulmonary fibrosis.
(b) Pleural calcification.
(c) Bronchial carcinoma.
(d) Progressive pulmonary function impairment after exposure has ceased.
(e) Premature greying of the hair.

2.52 The following drugs may cause pulmonary infiltration leading to fibrosis:
(a) Aspirin.
(b) Amiodarone.
(c) Busulphan.
(d) Cyclophosphamide.
(e) Oxprenolol.

2.53 The following are complications/risks involved with oxygen therapy:
(a) Retrolental fibroplasia in the elderly.
(b) Hypoventilation.
(c) Intra-alveolar haemorrhage.
(d) Fire.
(e) Pneumothorax.

2.54 An episode of acute severe asthma (status asthmaticus) is usually accompanied by:
(a) Bradycardia.
(b) Pulsus paradoxus.
(c) Low PO_2.
(d) Relative resistance to beta-2-adrenoceptor agonists.
(e) Pulsus alternans.

2.55 In asthmatics:
(a) Morning levels of plasma cortisol are low.
(b) Oral steroids should be reserved for status asthmaticus.
(c) Steroid aerosols should be used regularly in those requiring continuous oral steroids.
(d) Antibiotics should be prescribed for each acute exacerbation.
(e) Physical exercise should be limited.

2.51
(a)   TRUE
(b)   TRUE   – They are seen on chest X-ray and serve as a marker of previous exposure.
(c)   TRUE
(d)   TRUE   – Restrictive pulmonary defect.
(e)   FALSE

2.52
(a)   FALSE
(b)   TRUE
(c)   TRUE
(d)   TRUE
(e)   FALSE

2.53
(a)   FALSE   – This may occur with high concentration oxygen in the nenonatal period.
(b)   TRUE   – This occurs in the chronic bronchitic who relies on hypoxia as a ventilatory stimulus. Oxygen therapy should be given with care.
(c)   TRUE   – Occurs with prolonged exposure to oxygen concentrations in excess of 50%.
(d)   TRUE   – Oxygen is highly flammable.
(e)   FALSE

2.54
(a)   FALSE   – Tachycardia is the rule.
(b)   TRUE
(c)   TRUE
(d)   TRUE
(e)   FALSE   – This is a sign of left ventricular failure.

2.55
(a)   FALSE   – They are high as in normal people. Diurnal variations in asthma are not related to variation in cortisol levels.
(b)   FALSE   – Steroids should be used early with short high-dose courses if there is no response to other bronchodilators.
(c)   TRUE   – This reduces the oral maintenance dose.
(d)   FALSE   – Only if exacerbation is due to infection.
(e)   FALSE   – With optimal treatment asthmatics can lead normal lives.

2.56 Cigarette smoking increases the risk of developing:
(a) Adenocarcinoma of lung.
(b) Alveolar cell carcinoma of lung.
(c) Mesothelioma.
(d) Ischaemic heart disease.
(e) Emphysema.

2.57 Bronchiolitis:
(a) Is caused by a rhinovirus.
(b) Occurs most commonly in 1–3 year olds.
(c) May cause cot death.
(d) Produces widespread wheezes.
(e) Usually causes respiratory failure.

2.58 The following may produce pneumonia in those patients with acquired immune deficiency syndrome (AIDS):
(a) Cytomegalovirus.
(b) *Cryptococcus.*
(c) *Aspergillus.*
(d) Mycobacterium tuberculosis.
(e) *Clostridium difficile.*

2.59 The following are characteristic of a pulmonary embolus:
(a) Hypoxia.
(b) Hypercapnia.
(c) Pleuritic chest pain.
(d) Collapsing pulse.
(e) Raised jugular venous pressure.

2.60 The FEV_1:
(a) Is measured with a peak flow meter.
(b) Is reduced in asthma.
(c) Is increased in pulmonary fibrosis.
(d) Decreases with age.
(e) Is the volume of air expired in the first minute of a maximal forced expiration.

2.56

(a)	FALSE	– All other types of lung cancer are caused by smoking.
(b)	TRUE	
(c)	FALSE	
(d)	TRUE	
(e)	TRUE	

2.57

(a)	FALSE	– It is caused by the respiratory syncytial virus.
(b)	FALSE	– Commonest in 3–6 month olds.
(c)	TRUE	
(d)	TRUE	
(e)	FALSE	– Uncommon but sometimes ventilation is necessary.

2.58

(a)	TRUE	
(b)	TRUE	
(c)	TRUE	
(d)	TRUE	
(e)	FALSE	– Produces pseudomembranous colitis.

2.59

(a)	TRUE	– Type I respiratory failure.
(b)	FALSE	– This is normal or low.
(c)	TRUE	
(d)	FALSE	
(e)	TRUE	

2.60

(a)	FALSE	
(b)	TRUE	
(c)	FALSE	– It is reduced, usually in proportion to FVC.
(d)	TRUE	
(e)	FALSE	– It is the volume expired in the first *second* of a maximal forced expiration.

3 Rheumatology

3.1 The following characteristically produce a symmetrical polyarthritis:
(a) Osteoarthritis.
(b) Rheumatoid arthritis.
(c) Systemic lupus erythematosus.
(d) Reiter's syndrome.
(e) Crohn's disease.

3.2 Involvement of the following articular regions are characteristic of rheumatoid arthritis:
(a) Distal interphalangeal joints.
(b) Proximal interphalangeal joints.
(c) Metacarpophalangeal joints.
(d) Lumbar spine.
(e) Knee joints.

3.3 The following are radiographic appearances associated with rheumatoid arthritis:
(a) Marginal erosions.
(b) Juxta-articular osteoporosis.
(c) Increase in joint space.
(d) Osteophyte formation.
(e) Subluxation.

3.4 Regarding systemic lupus erythematosus (SLE):
(a) It is commoner in men.
(b) Photosensitivity may occur.
(c) Complement (C3 and C4) levels are increased.
(d) Renal involvement is a good prognostic feature.
(e) The antinuclear factor is usually negative.

3.5 The following drugs may produce an SLE syndrome:
(a) Hydralazine.
(b) Aspirin.
(c) Procainamide.
(d) Phenytoin.
(e) Ranitidine.

3.1
(a)   FALSE   – This is usually oligoarticular. A hereditary polyarticular forms is seen in females.
(b)   TRUE
(c)   TRUE   – Sometimes indistinguishable from early rheumatoid arthritis.
(d)   FALSE   – Usually asymmetrical and affects lower limb joints.
(e)   FALSE   – Usually monoarticular affecting the larger lower limb joints.

3.2
(a)   FALSE   – Usually spared.
(b)   TRUE
(c)   TRUE
(d)   FALSE   – The cervical spine is often affected.
(e)   TRUE   – Larger synovial joints of limbs are commonly involved.

3.3
(a)   TRUE   – These are an indication for early specific treatment.
(b)   TRUE   – Occurs early.
(c)   FALSE   – There is loss of joint space with destruction
(d)   FALSE   – These occur in osteoarthritis.
(e)   TRUE

3.4
(a)   FALSE   – 90% of cases occur in women aged 20–40 years.
(b)   TRUE
(c)   FALSE   – These are usually reduced.
(d)   FALSE   – Renal involvement occurs in 50% cases and is a bad prognostic feature (50% 5 year survival).
(e)   FALSE   – It is positive in over 95% of cases.

3.5
(a)   TRUE   – Drug induced lupus differs from true SLE as follows: (1) renal disease is rare, (2) DNA antibodies are not characteristic, (3) sex incidence is equal, and (4) regression with drug withdrawal.
(b)   FALSE
(c)   TRUE
(d)   TRUE
(e)   FALSE

3.6 **The following are clinical features of SLE:**
(a) Depression.
(b) Alopecia.
(c) Pleural effusions.
(d) Extra-articular nodules.
(e) Uveitis.

3.7 **The following may produce hyperuricaemia:**
(a) Pregnancy.
(b) Renal failure.
(c) Wilson's disease.
(d) Polycythaemia rubra vera.
(e) Obesity.

3.8 **The following drugs are used in acute gout:**
(a) Indomethacin.
(b) Allopurinol.
(c) Colchicine.
(d) Probenecid.
(e) Aspirin.

3.9 **Regarding polymyalgia rheumatica:**
(a) It is commoner in women.
(b) The ESR is usually less than 30 mm/h.
(c) It is associated with weakness of the limb girdle muscles.
(d) Weight loss may occur.
(e) There is a risk of blindness developing if untreated.

3.10 **Gout:**
(a) Is associated with calcium pyrophosphate crystals deposited in the cartilage.
(b) May cause subcutaneous nodules on the pinnae of the ears.
(c) Is associated with HLA B27.
(d) Commonly involves the first metatarsophalangeal joint.
(e) May result in chronic renal failure.

3.6
(a)   TRUE   –   Two-thirds of patients develop CNS involvement including chorea, myelitis and convulsions.
(b)   TRUE   –   Occurs in 60% of cases.
(c)   TRUE
(d)   FALSE
(e)   FALSE   –   This is a feature of rheumatoid disease.

3.7
(a)   FALSE   –   Associated with low serum urate.
(b)   TRUE   –   Elimination of uric acid is mainly renal.
(c)   FALSE   –   Associated with low serum urate.
(d)   TRUE   –   Due to increased formation of uric acid.
(e)   TRUE   –   Mechanism uncertain.

3.8
(a)   TRUE
(b)   FALSE   –   Used in long-term management.
(c)   TRUE   –   Used for short courses. Nausea and diarrhoea are relatively common side-effects.
(d)   FALSE   –   Used in long-term management. It is a uricosuric agent.
(e)   FALSE   –   It may precipitate acute gout.

3.9
(a)   TRUE
(b)   FALSE   –   ESR is usually high (> 70 mm/h)
(c)   FALSE   –   There is no weakness or wasting; usually stiffness.
(d)   TRUE
(e)   TRUE   –   It is associated with temporal arteritis and requires treatment with steroids.

3.10
(a)   FALSE   –   This occurs in pseudogout.
(b)   TRUE   –   These gouty tophi are deposits of urate and can occur elsewhere in subcutaneous tissues.
(c)   FALSE
(d)   TRUE   –   This is affected in first attack in 75% of cases.
(e)   TRUE   –   Due to chronic urate nephropathy if untreated.

3.11 Pseudogout:
(a) Is more common in females than gout.
(b) Most commonly presents with arthralgia involving the ankle.
(c) Produces joint effusions which contain calcium pyrophosphate crystals.
(d) Is associated with calcification of joint cartilage.
(e) Is associated with haemochromatosis.

3.12 Rheumatoid factor:
(a) Is an immunoglobulin of the IgG class.
(b) Is an antibody to IgG.
(c) Is present in the serum if rheumatoid nodules are present.
(d) May be present in the absence of rheumatoid arthritis.
(e) Is usually present in psoriatic arthropathy.

3.13 The following are associated with a poor prognosis in rheumatoid arthritis:
(a) Acute onset.
(b) Bone erosions on X-ray.
(c) Subcutaneous nodules.
(d) Low ESR.
(e) Extra-articular manifestations.

3.14 Chloroquine:
(a) Is effective in treating psoriatic arthropathy.
(b) Is used in the treatment of SLE.
(c) Is used in the treatment of malaria.
(d) May cause retinal damage.
(e) Is used as a second line treatment in rheumatoid arthritis.

3.15 The following are side-effects of gold therapy:
(a) Membranous glomerulonephritis.
(b) Hypertension.
(c) Thrombocytopenia.
(d) Polycythaemia.
(e) Neutropenia.

3.11
(a)	TRUE	– Ratio male : female is 2 : 1. In gout it is 6 : 1.
(b)	FALSE	
(c)	TRUE	– These are positively birefringent in polarized light whereas sodium urate crystals are negatively birefringent.
(d)	TRUE	
(e)	TRUE	– Also associated with diabetes mellitus, hyperparathyroidism and chronic renal failure.

3.12
(a)	FALSE	– It is an IgM immunoglobulin.
(b)	TRUE	– It is an autoantibody.
(c)	TRUE	
(d)	TRUE	– It occurs in 4% of the general population and rises with age.
(e)	FALSE	

3.13
(a)	FALSE	– Insidious onset is associated with a poor prognosis.
(b)	TRUE	
(c)	TRUE	
(d)	FALSE	– Raised ESR is associated with a poor prognosis.
(e)	TRUE	

3.14
(a)	FALSE	– It should be avoided as it may precipitate exfoliation.
(b)	TRUE	
(c)	TRUE	
(d)	TRUE	– This may be irreversible and patients require monitoring by an opthalmologist.
(e)	TRUE	

3.15
(a)	TRUE	– Presents as proteinuria in 10%.
(b)	FALSE	– Hypotension due to vasodilatation may occur acutely following dose.
(c)	TRUE	
(d)	FALSE	
(e)	TRUE	

3.16 The following are associated with Felty's syndrome:
(a) Hepatomegaly.
(b) Splenomegaly.
(c) Leg ulcers.
(d) Asymmetrical arthropathy.
(e) Lymphadenopathy.

3.17 Psoriatic arthritis:
(a) May be clinically indistinguishable from rheumatoid arthritis.
(b) Is associated with subcutaneous nodules.
(c) Is associated with nail pitting.
(d) May respond to gold therapy.
(e) Is associated with pleural effusions.

3.18 The following are characteristic of osteoarthritis:
(a) Heberden's nodes.
(b) Heliotrope rash around the eyes.
(c) Bouchard's nodes
(d) Raised ESR.
(e) Early morning stiffness.

3.19 The following are associated with the antigen HLA B27:
(a) Rheumatoid arthritis.
(b) A region in the sixth chromosome.
(c) Ankylosing spondylitis.
(d) Psoriatic spondylitis.
(e) Coeliac disease.

3.20 Behcet's syndrome:
(a) Is commoner in females.
(b) Is associated with arthralgia of the small joints.
(c) Characteristically involves mouth ulcers.
(d) Is associated with HLA B8.
(e) Is rare in Japan.

3.16

(a)	FALSE	
(b)	TRUE	– This results in hypersplenism with anaemia, leucopenia and thrombocytopenia.
(c)	TRUE	– These are due to vasculitis.
(d)	FALSE	– It is a syndrome which includes rheumatoid arthritis.
(e)	TRUE	

3.17

(a)	TRUE	– In 30% of cases.
(b)	FALSE	
(c)	TRUE	
(d)	TRUE	
(e)	FALSE	

3.18

(a)	TRUE	– These are due to osteophytes at the distal interphalangeal joints and are usually symmetrical.
(b)	FALSE	– This is characteristic of dermatomyositis.
(c)	TRUE	– As for Heberden's nodes but at proximal interphalangeal joints.
(d)	FALSE	
(e)	FALSE	– Pain and loss of function occur. Stiffness uncommon but may be present if there is an inflammatory component.

3.19

(a)	FALSE	– Associated with HLA DRW4.
(b)	TRUE	– The inheritence of the 'human leucocyte A antigens' is controlled by a small region on the sixth chromosome.
(c)	TRUE	– It is present in 96% of patients (compared with 7% of the general population).
(d)	TRUE	
(e)	FALSE	– Associated with HLA B8 and DRW 3.

3.20

(a)	FALSE	– It is twice as common in males.
(b)	FALSE	– Large joints are usually involved.
(c)	TRUE	
(d)	FALSE	– It is associated with HLA B5.
(e)	FALSE	– It is more common in Japan and Eastern Mediterranean countries compared with Western Europe.

3.21 **The following are recognized side-effects of non-steroidal anti-inflammatory drugs:**
(a) Inappropriate ADH secretion.
(b) Renal papillary necrosis.
(c) Hepatic encephalopathy.
(d) Fluid retention.
(e) Angiodysplasia of the stomach.

3.22 **The following are associated with ankylosing spondylitis:**
(a) Pulmonary fibrosis.
(b) Aortic stenosis.
(c) Iritis.
(d) An autosomal recessive inheritance pattern.
(e) Secondary amyloidosis.

3.23 **Reiter's disease:**
(a) May follow *Campylobacter* enteritis.
(b) Is associated with a polyarticular asymmetrical arthritis affecting large joints of the lower limbs.
(c) Is common in negroes.
(d) May involve conjunctivitis.
(e) Is associated with keratoderma blennorrhagica.

3.24 **The following may lead to joint laxity:**
(a) Marfan's syndrome.
(b) Ehlers–Danlos syndrome.
(c) Down's syndrome.
(d) Sarcoidosis.
(e) Turner's syndrome.

3.25 **The following may exacerbate systemic lupus erythematosus:**
(a) Oral contraceptive pill.
(b) Red wine.
(c) Acute coryza.
(d) Sunlight.
(e) Prednisolone.

3.21
(a)   FALSE
(b)   TRUE
(c)   FALSE
(d)   TRUE
(e)   FALSE

3.22
(a)   TRUE   – This may be progressive and fatal.
(b)   FALSE – Aortic regurgitation occurs due to aortitis.
(c)   TRUE
(d)   FALSE – It is related to HLA B27. The probability of the off-
                spring of an HLA B27-positive patient developing the
                disease is 5–10%.
(e)   TRUE   – Occurs in 6% of cases in the later stage of the
                disease.

3.23
(a)   TRUE   – It is a post-infectious syndrome. May follow *Shigella*,
                Salmonella and *Yersinia* infection as well as chlamydial
                infection.
(b)   TRUE   – Usually affects small and large joints.
(c)   FALSE – The HLA B27 antigen is uncommon in Negroes.
(d)   TRUE   – In 30% of cases.
(e)   TRUE   – This is a pustular hyperkeratotic rash involving the soles
                of the feet and palms of the hands. It occurs in 15%
                of cases.

3.24
(a)   TRUE
(b)   TRUE
(c)   TRUE
(d)   FALSE – Produces a migratory, non-destructive, symmetrical
                polyarthritis.
(e)   FALSE

3.25
(a)   TRUE
(b)   FALSE
(c)   TRUE   – It can be exacerbated by any infection.
(d)   TRUE
(e)   FALSE – Steroids are used in the treatment.

3.26 **Regarding septic arthritis:**
(a) *E. coli* is the most common infecting organism.
(b) It is usually polyarticular.
(c) It is more common in the presence of rheumatoid arthritis.
(d) Joint aspiration is contraindicated.
(e) It is best treated with intra-articular antibiotics.

3.27 **Systemic sclerosis:**
(a) Is commoner in females.
(b) Has a worse prognosis in Caucasians than Negroes.
(c) Results in excessive production of collagen by fibroblasts.
(d) Is diagnosed in the presence of clinical features and a positive rheumatoid factor.
(e) In the presence of a positive antinuclear factor antibody, is diagnostic.

3.28 **The following are clinical features of systemic sclerosis:**
(a) Hyperpigmentation of the skin.
(b) Steatorrhoea.
(c) Sacroileitis.
(d) Malar rash.
(e) Subcutaneous emphysema.

3.29 **The following are associated with a poor prognosis in systemic sclerosis:**
(a) Onset in the young (< 40 years).
(b) Pulmonary fibrosis.
(c) Sclerodactyly.
(d) Renal involvement.
(e) Trunk involvement.

3.30 **Polyarteritis nodosa:**
(a) Is associated with an abdominal aortic aneurysm.
(b) May cause pulmonary eosinophilia.
(c) Has an excellent prognosis.
(d) Is associated with an arthropathy indistinguishable from that in rheumatoid arthritis.
(e) May present with a myocardial infarction.

3.26
(a)	FALSE	– *Staphylococcus aureus* is the commonest pathogen.
(b)	FALSE	– Usually a single joint is effected.
(c)	TRUE	
(d)	FALSE	– This is essential to make a microbiological diagnosis. It also relieves pain and repeat aspirations are indicated.
(e)	FALSE	– Bactericidal levels of antibiotics are reached in the synovial fluid after systemic administration. Antibiotics are usually continued for 6 weeks.

3.27
(a)	TRUE	– Ratio is 15 : 1 under 45 years and 2 : 1 (female : male) over this age.
(b)	FALSE	
(c)	TRUE	
(d)	FALSE	– Rheumatoid factor is positive in 30% of cases.
(e)	FALSE	– There is no specific test. Antinuclear factor in a nucleolar pattern and antibody against a nuclear protein Scl–70 are particularly associated with this disorder.

3.28
(a)	TRUE	– Vitiligo may also occur.
(b)	TRUE	– Due to malabsorption caused by gut hypomotility and secondary bacterial overgrowth.
(c)	FALSE	
(d)	FALSE	– This is characteristic of SLE.
(e)	FALSE	– Subcutaneous calcification may occur.

3.29
(a)	FALSE	– Poor prognosis if older at onset.
(b)	TRUE	
(c)	FALSE	– Also patients with CREST syndrome have a better prognosis than those with diffuse scleroderma.
(d)	TRUE	
(e)	TRUE	

3.30
(a)	FALSE	– There is fibrinoid necrosis of the media of small and medium sized arteries. Healing by fibrosis causes small aneurysms.
(b)	TRUE	– Asthma may occur.
(c)	FALSE	– Five year survival is 40%
(d)	FALSE	– Associated with a non-deforming polyarthritis mainly affecting the lower limbs.
(e)	TRUE	

3.31 Sjorgen's syndrome:
(a) Is associated with a positive rheumatoid factor.
(b) Is associated with dry eyes and mouth.
(c) May be associated with rheumatoid arthritis.
(d) Is commoner in men.
(e) Is associated with infertility.

3.32 The following are associated with Paget's disease of bone:
(a) Raised serum alkaline phosphatase.
(b) Reduced urinary hydroxyproline.
(c) Optic atrophy.
(d) Raised serum uric acid.
(e) Deafness.

3.33 Sulphasalazine:
(a) Is ineffective in rheumatoid arthritis.
(b) Is effective in inflammatory bowel disease.
(c) May cause infertility in the male.
(d) May cause neutropenia.
(e) Is the first drug of choice in psoriatic arthropathy.

3.34 Polymyositis:
(a) Is associated with HLA B8.
(b) Is associated with an elevated serum lactate dehydrogenase.
(c) Is treated with non-steroidal anti-inflammatory drugs in the first instance.
(d) Causes a proximal myopathy.
(e) Is commoner in men.

3.35 The Shoulder–Hand Syndrome:
(a) Is due to irritation of autonomic pathways.
(b) May occur following appendicitis.
(c) May occur following a stroke.
(d) May occur following a myocardial infarction.
(e) Is uncommon in Scotland.

3.31

(a)	TRUE	– Positive in 100% of cases.
(b)	TRUE	– Due to reduced secretions from lachrimal and salivary glands (sicca syndrome).
(c)	TRUE	– 50% of cases are associated with rheumatoid arthritis.
(d)	FALSE	– Commoner in women (9 : 1).
(e)	FALSE	

3.32

(a)	TRUE	
(b)	FALSE	– It is increased.
(c)	TRUE	– Due to compression of optic nerve. There may also be angioid streaks in the retina.
(d)	TRUE	
(e)	TRUE	

3.33

(a)	FALSE	
(b)	TRUE	
(c)	TRUE	– It is reversible on withdrawal.
(d)	TRUE	
(e)	FALSE	

3.34

(a)	TRUE	– It is also associated with viruses (rubella, influenza, coxsackie), other connective tissue disorders and underlying malignancy.
(b)	TRUE	– Skeletal muscle enzymes aldolase and/or creatine phosphokinase are also elevated.
(c)	FALSE	– Early treatment with high-dose prednisolone (40–60 mg once daily) is indicated. If no response after 2 months azathioprine or methotrexate is used.
(d)	TRUE	
(e)	FALSE	– Commoner in women (3 : 1).

3.35

(a)	TRUE	– Some patients benefit from cervical sympathectomy and others respond to steroids.
(b)	FALSE	
(c)	TRUE	
(d)	TRUE	– It may also follow injuries and burns of the arm.
(e)	FALSE	

The patient develops pain in the shoulder and hand. Movements are painful and muscle atrophy may occur.

3.36 The following may complicate rheumatoid arthritis:
(a) Amyloidosis.
(b) Mononeuritis multiplex.
(c) Premature greying of the hair.
(d) Tophi formation.
(e) Cataracts.

3.37 The following are radiological features of gout:
(a) Ankylosis.
(b) New bone formation.
(c) Osteoporosis.
(d) Erosions.
(e) Soft tissue swelling.

3.38 Regarding osteoporosis:
(a) It is associated with a raised serum alkaline phosphatase.
(b) It is more common in women under 40 years than older women.
(c) Progression can be reduced with hormone replacement therapy.
(d) Urinary calcium is increased.
(e) It may be associated with vertebral fractures.

3.39 The following are associated with rheumatoid disease:
(a) Low serum albumin.
(b) High serum globulin.
(c) High serum alkaline phosphatase.
(d) High serum iron.
(e) Low C-reactive protein.

3.40 Regarding fourth lumbar nerve root involvement in postero-lateral disc protrusion:
(a) Sensory changes occur on the lateral aspect of foot and ankle.
(b) There is weakness of foot inversion.
(c) Knee jerk is diminished or absent.
(d) Ankle jerk is diminished or absent.
(e) There is weakness of knee extension.

3.36
(a) TRUE – The incidence is 5–10%.
(b) TRUE – Particularly of the digital nerves, ulnar nerves and lateral popliteal nerves.
(c) FALSE – This may complicate chloroquine therapy.
(d) FALSE – These occur in chronic gout.
(e) FALSE – This may be a complication of steroid therapy.

3.37
(a) FALSE
(b) FALSE
(c) TRUE – This is a later manifestation.
(d) TRUE – These occur at the joint margins and are caused by deposition of sodium biurate in bone.
(e) TRUE – Those caused by tophi are asymmetrical and become calcified late in the disease.

3.38
(a) FALSE
(b) FALSE – Commoner in post-menopausal women as oestrogens have a protective effect.
(c) TRUE
(d) FALSE – There are no biochemical abnormalities.
(e) TRUE – Vertebral fractures, Colles fractures and fractured neck of femur are common presentation.

3.39
(a) TRUE – This is due to increased catabolism.
(b) TRUE
(c) TRUE
(d) FALSE – It is always low due to inflammatory activity and serum total iron binding capacity is normal or low.
(e) FALSE – Similar to ESR but preferable as it responds more quickly to changes in inflammatory activity.

3.40
(a) FALSE – This occurs in first sacral nerve root involvement. Medial aspects of calf and shin is affected.
(b) TRUE
(c) TRUE
(d) FALSE
(e) TRUE

3.41 **The following are associated with carpal tunnel syndrome:**
(a) Phenytoin.
(b) Osteoarthritis.
(c) Rheumatoid arthritis.
(d) Hypothyroidism.
(e) Acromegaly.

3.42 **Regarding intra-articular steroid injections:**
(a) They may be repeated frequently with no ill effects.
(b) Septic arthritis is a common complication.
(c) Prednisolone is most commonly used.
(d) They should never be used if there is any evidence of septic arthritis.
(e) They are effective in suppressing the inflammatory reaction of the synovial membrane.

3.43 **The following are ideal features of an armchair designed for an arthritic patient:**
(a) High almost upright backrest.
(b) Low seat to floor height.
(c) Soft seat cushion.
(d) Wooden armrests with no protruding ends.
(e) Wheels on all legs.

3.44 **The following may cause a proximal myopathy:**
(a) Prednisolone.
(b) Osteoporosis.
(c) Osteomalacia.
(d) Acromegaly.
(e) Polymyalgia Rheumatica.

3.45 **The following are recognized features of osteomalacia:**
(a) Bone pain.
(b) Waddling gait.
(c) Reduced serum alkaline phosphatase.
(d) Decreased serum alkaline phosphatase.
(e) Looser's zones.

3.41
(a)	FALSE
(b)	TRUE
(c)	TRUE
(d)	TRUE
(e)	TRUE

3.42

(a)   FALSE   – This may give rise to destructive changes within the joint.

(b)   FALSE   – The risk is low if aseptic facilities are used which is mandatory.

(c)   FALSE   – Hydrocortisone, Triamcinolone and Methylprednisolone are all widely used.

(d)   TRUE

(e)   TRUE

3.43

(a)   TRUE   – This supports the whole spine and the head.

(b)   FALSE   – This should be high to allow easier standing.

(c)   FALSE   – This should be firm.

(d)   FALSE   – These should be padded for comfort and should have protruding ends to hold onto when standing.

(e)   FALSE   – This may cause accidents.

3.44
(a)	TRUE
(b)	FALSE
(c)	TRUE
(d)	TRUE
(e)	FALSE – There is no weakness.

3.45

(a)   TRUE   – There is also tenderness. May present as generalized aches and pains in the elderly.

(b)   TRUE   – Due to myopathy affecting the hip girdle muscles.

(c)   FALSE   – It is increased.

(d)   FALSE   – It is increased.

(e)   TRUE   – These are pseudofractures (Milkman fractures) best seen in the pubic rami, necks of humerus and femur and outer border of the scapula. There may also be pathological fractures.

3.46 **The following are risk factors for osteoporosis:**
(a) Smoking.
(b) Exercise.
(c) Obesity.
(d) Thyrotoxicosis.
(e) Negroid ethnic origin.

3.47 **Regarding Paget's disease of bone:**
(a) It may be asymptomatic.
(b) There is decrease bone resorption.
(c) Osteoarthritis is more common.
(d) Non-steroidal anti-inflammatory drugs slow down the progression of the disease.
(e) It is commoner in males.

3.48 **Regarding Dupuytren's contracture:**
(a) It is usually associated with asymmetrical polyarthritis.
(b) There is a genetic link.
(c) It is commoner in women.
(d) The incidence increases with age.
(e) It is more common in diabetics.

3.49 **Rheumatoid factor is usually positive in the following:**
(a) Rheumatoid arthritis with subcutaneous nodules.
(b) Ankylosing spondylitis.
(c) Osteoarthritis.
(d) Psoriatic arthritis.
(e) Sjorgren's syndrome.

3.50 **The following are associated with human leucocyte antigen (HLA) DR3:**
(a) Sjorgren's syndrome. ✓
(b) Myasthenia gravis. ✓
(c) Rheumatoid arthritis. DRw 4
(d) Osteoarthritis.
(e) Systemic lupus erythematosus. ✓

3.46
(a)   TRUE
(b)   FALSE   –   Lack of exercise is a risk factor.
(c)   TRUE
(d)   TRUE
(e)   FALSE   –   It is more common in Caucasians.

3.47
(a)   TRUE   –   Only in 5–10% of cases is it clinically important. It
occurs in 1% of the population over 50 years.
(b)   FALSE   –   This is increased.
(c)   TRUE
(d)   FALSE   –   They are used for symptomatic pain relief.
(e)   TRUE

3.48
(a)   FALSE   –   It is a condition resulting in thickening of the palmar
fascia with resultant flexion contractures of the fourth
and fifth fingers.
(b)   TRUE
(c)   FALSE
(d)   TRUE
(e)   TRUE

3.49
(a)   TRUE
(b)   FALSE
(c)   FALSE
(d)   FALSE
(e)   TRUE

3.50
(a)   TRUE
(b)   TRUE
(c)   FALSE   –   Associated with DRW4.
(d)   FALSE
(e)   TRUE

3.51 **Regarding immune reactions:**
(a) Type III reaction is involved in rheumatoid disease.
(b) Type IV is mediated by T cells.
(c) Type II reaction is complement dependent.
(d) Type I is IgG mediated.
(e) Type V is IgG mediated.

3.52 **Regerding mixed connective tissue disease (MCTD):**
(a) It is an overlap syndrome combining features of SLE, scleroderma and polymyostis.
(b) Antibodies to nuclear ribonucleoprotein (nRNp) are usually present.
(c) The prognosis is poor.
(d) Renal disease is common.
(e) Antibodies to double stranded DNA are present.

3.53 **Regarding osteoarthrosis:**
(a) It is commoner in West African countries.
(b) It is commoner in women.
(c) Knee joint involvement is rare.
(d) There is destruction of articular cartilage.
(e) It occurs prematurely in alkaptonuria.

3.54 **Raynaud's phenomenon is a recognized feature of:**
(a) Polymyositis.
(b) Polyarteritis nodosa.
(c) Systemic lupus erythematosus.
(d) Temporal arteritis.
(e) Scleroderma.

3.55 **The following are second line drugs used in the treatment of rheumatoid arthritis:**
(a) Indomethecin.
(b) Penicillamine.
(c) Prednisolone.
(d) Gold.
(e) Chloroquine.

3.51

(a)	TRUE	–	This involves the deposition of an immune complex (antigen and antibody) in tissues leading to inflammation.
(b)	TRUE	–	Delayed hypersensitivity.
(c)	TRUE	–	This is the cytotoxic reaction, e.g. autoimmune haemolytic anaemia. Type III is complement dependent.
(d)	FALSE	–	It Is IgE mediated.
(e)	TRUE		

3.52

(a)	TRUE		
(b)	TRUE		
(c)	FALSE	–	Responds to steroids and prognosis is good.
(d)	FALSE	–	It is rare.
(e)	FALSE	–	This is characteristic of SLE.

3.53

(a)	FALSE	–	It is very common in West Africa.
(b)	TRUE		
(c)	FALSE		
(d)	TRUE		
(e)	TRUE	–	In this condition there is a genetically determined absence of homogentisic acid oxidase so that homogentisic acid accumulates in cartilage causing atrophy and osteoarthrosis.

3.54

(a)	TRUE	–	Occurs in 30% of cases.
(b)	FALSE		
(c)	TRUE	–	Occurs in 10%.
(d)	FALSE		
(e)	TRUE		

3.55

(a)	FALSE	–	This is a non-steroidal anti-inflammatory drug and is used as a first-line agent. Unlike second and third line drugs it does not influence the underlying disease process.
(b)	TRUE		
(c)	FALSE	–	Corticosteroids and immunosuppressant cytotoxic drugs are used as third line therapy.
(d)	TRUE		
(e)	TRUE		

3.56 Regarding the CREST syndrome:
(a) An antinuclear antibody with specificity for a component of the chromosomal centromere is present in the serum.
(b) Dysphagia is a symptom.
(c) Raynaud's phenomenon is uncommon.
(d) The prognosis is poor.
(e) Gangrene may occur.

3.57 The following are radiological changes in psoriatic arthritis:
(a) Ligamentous ossification in the spine.
(b) Absorption of tufts of distal phalanges.
(c) Subcutaneous calcification.
(d) Osteophytes.
(e) Erosions at joint margins.

3.58 Regarding gonococcal arthritis:
(a) It is usually a symmetrical polyarthritis.
(b) The onset is insidious.
(c) The organisms are always isolated from synovial fluid.
(d) It is commoner in women.
(e) Tetracycline is the drug of choice.

3.59 The following are recognized associations of psoriatic arthritis:
(a) Onycholysis.
(b) HLA DR3.
(c) Pulmonary fibrosis.
(d) Sacroiliitis.
(e) Finger clubbing.

3.60 The following are features of Whipple's disease:
(a) Vitiligo.
(b) Malabsorption.
(c) Sacroiliitis.
(d) Isolation of streptococci from synovial fluid.
(e) Response to tetracycline.

3.56

(a)   TRUE   – This is a useful diagnostic and prognostic aid.
(b)   TRUE   – Due to oesophageal immotility and stricture formation.
(c)   FALSE
(d)   FALSE – It is more favourable than systemic sclerosis.
(e)   TRUE   – Due to severe peripheral vasospasm.

3.57

(a)   TRUE
(b)   TRUE
(c)   FALSE
(d)   FALSE
(e)   TRUE   – Changes are similar to those in rheumatoid arthritis. Osteoporosis is not a pronounced feature.

3.58

(a)   FALSE – It is asymmetrical and migratory.
(b)   FALSE – It is usually acute.
(c)   FALSE – Only in 20% of cases.
(d)   TRUE
(e)   FALSE – Penicillin is the drug of choice and should be continued for at least 2 weeks.

3.59

(a)   TRUE   – This is elevation of the nail from the nail bed which is a feature of psoriasis.
(b)   FALSE – It is associated with HLA B27.
(c)   FALSE
(d)   TRUE
(e)   FALSE

3.60

(a)   FALSE – There is usually skin pigmentation.
(b)   TRUE
(c)   TRUE   – There may also be a non-erosive, migratory polyarthritis which is more common.
(d)   FALSE – Unidentified rod shaped organisms can be isolated from the lamina propria and the synovial membrane.
(e)   TRUE   – Usually given in a dose of 1 g daily for 1 year.

4 Infectious diseases

4.1 The following are RNA viruses:
(a) Influenza A.
(b) Coxsackie.
(c) Cytomegalovirus.
(d) Epstein–Barr virus.
(e) Measles.

4.2 Herpes simplex virus infection:
(a) Can produce an encephalitis which runs a benign course.
(b) Of the genitalia may be passed to the newborn with fatal consequences.
(c) Type 2 is implicated in cervical cancer.
(d) Causes chickenpox.
(e) Causes 'cold sores'.

4.3 The following are characterized by an erythematous maculo-papular or petechial rash:
(a) Meningococcal infection.
(b) Rubella.
(c) Chickenpox.
(d) Malaria.
(e) Scarlet fever.

4.4 Scabies:
(a) Has an incubation period of 3 months.
(b) Is transmitted by droplet infection.
(c) Produces a rash most commonly seen on the scalp.
(d) May be complicated by secondary infection.
(e) Is treated with 1% gamma benzene hexachloride.

4.5 Regarding gentamicin:
(a) It is a penicillin.
(b) It is bacteriostatic.
(c) It is active against most Gram-negative organisms.
(d) Plasma levels must be monitored to avoid toxicity.
(e) It may cause deafness.

4.1
(a) TRUE
(b) TRUE
(c) FALSE – DNA virus (Herpes virus).
(d) FALSE – DNA virus (Herpes virus).
(e) TRUE

4.2
(a) FALSE – Herpes encephalitis is a severe condition with a high mortality (60%).
(b) TRUE – Presents a few days after birth with vomiting, convulsions and circulatory collapse.
(c) TRUE
(d) FALSE – This is caused by the varicella-zoster virus which is also a Herpes virus.
(e) TRUE

4.3
(a) TRUE
(b) TRUE
(c) FALSE – Produces a papulovesicular or blisteriform rash.
(d) FALSE
(e) TRUE

4.4
(a) FALSE – Incubation period is 1–3 weeks.
(b) FALSE – The parasite *Sarcoptes scabiei* which causes scabies is transmitted by close bodily contact.
(c) FALSE – The scalp is usually spared. The papular, intensely itchy rash is most common on the wrists and between the fingers but also involves the trunk and limbs.
(d) TRUE – This is the most serious complication.
(e) TRUE – This is applied to the body after a bath. The patient bathes again the following day. All contacts should be treated and all clothes and bedlinen laundered.

4.5
(a) FALSE – It is an aminoglycoside.
(b) FALSE – It is bacteriocidal.
(c) TRUE – It is active against staphylococci but streptococci tend to be resistant.
(d) TRUE
(e) TRUE – Eighth nerve damage and nephrotoxicity are the two major side-effects of this drug.

4.6 **Regarding cytomegalovirus (CMV) infection:**
(a) The majority of adults are immune.
(b) It may produce hepatitis.
(c) If acquired during pregnancy it is harmless to the fetus.
(d) It may produce a glandular fever like illness.
(e) It may produce a pneumonitis in the immunosuppressed due to reactivation of the virus.

4.7 **The following diseases may be caused by the Epstein–Barr virus:**
(a) Nasopharyngeal carcinoma.
(b) Whooping cough.
(c) Glandular fever.
(d) Burkitt's lymphoma.
(e) Dysentry.

4.8 **Glandular fever:**
(a) Produces a hypersensitive reaction to ampicillin.
(b) Is associated with atypical red cells in the peripheral blood.
(c) Rarely causes a lymphadenopathy.
(d) May be mimicked by toxoplasmosis.
(e) May cause swelling of the lachrymal gland.

4.9 **The following are recognized features of glandular fever:**
(a) Hepatitis.
(b) Myocarditis.
(c) Retinitis.
(d) Haemolytic anaemia.
(e) Hemiparesis.

4.10 **Acylclovir:**
(a) Is active against myxoviruses.
(b) May be given intravenously.
(c) Levels in serum may be increased by probenecid.
(d) Prevents the development of post-herpetic neuralgia.
(e) Commonly precipitates severe depression.

4.6
(a) TRUE – 60-90% have antibodies to CMV.
(b) TRUE
(c) FALSE – 10% suffer from significant brain damage. It may cause microcephaly, chorioretinitis and cerebral calcification. It causes significant mental retardation in 400 births per year in the UK.
(d) TRUE
(e) TRUE

4.7
(a) TRUE
(b) FALSE – This is caused by *Bordetella pertussis*.
(c) TRUE
(d) TRUE
(e) FALSE – This is caused by *Entamoeba histolytica* or organisms of the *Shigella* group.

4.8
(a) TRUE – This causes a severe maculopapular rash and should be avoided.
(b) FALSE – Atypical monoctyes are present (infectious mononucleosis).
(c) FALSE – Lymphadenopathy occurs in almost all cases.
(d) TRUE
(e) TRUE

4.9
(a) TRUE – A large number of cases are associated with a raised alanine aminotransferase. Less commonly the jaundice may be cholestatic. It is often subclinical.
(b) TRUE
(c) FALSE
(d) TRUE
(e) FALSE

4.10
(a) FALSE – It is active against herpes virus, in particular Herpes simplex and Varicella-zoster. It is effective only if started at the onset of infection.
(b) TRUE
(c) TRUE – Probenecid reduces excretion of acyclovir.
(d) FALSE – useful in acute herpes zoster.
(e) FALSE

4.11 **Regarding chickenpox:**
(a) It is associated with a papulovesicular rash which is peripherally distributed.
(b) The illness is milder in the adult.
(c) Vaccination is reducing the incidence.
(d) It may occur in the young after contact with a patient who has shingles.
(e) It may be complicated by encephalitis.

4.12 **Herpes zoster:**
(a) Is commoner in the young.
(b) Is usually bilateral in distribution.
(c) May cause permanent scarring.
(d) Pain and paraesthesia may persist for months.
(e) May be recurrent.

4.13 **The following organisms are Gram-negative:**
(a) *Neisseria meningitidis.*
(b) *Haemophilus influenzae.*
(c) *Staphylococcus aureus.*
(d) *Streptococcus faecalis.*
(e) Hepatitis A.

4.14 **Regarding bacterial meningitis:**
(a) *Escherichia coli* is the usual pathogen in the elderly.
(b) Kernig's sign is usually negative.
(c) Benzylpenicillin is the antibiotic of choice for *Haemophilus infuenzae* meningitis.
(d) Petechial rash commonly accompanies meningococcal meningitis.
(e) The CSF sugar is usually > 10 mmol/l.

4.15 **The following are recognized complications of bacterial meningitis:**
(a) Deafness.
(b) Bell's Palsy.
(c) Hydrocephalus.
(d) Destructive progressive polyarthritis.
(e) Epilepsy.

4.11

(a)	FALSE	– The rash is mainly central.
(b)	FALSE	– Adults have a more severe illness with systemic upset and pneumonitis.
(c)	TRUE	
(d)	TRUE	– Herpes zoster is caused by the varicella-zoster virus. After an attack of chickenpox the virus persists in the sensory and dorsal root ganglia. If reactivated shingles occurs. Shingles does not develop from contact with chickenpox.
(e)	TRUE	– Usually takes the form of a cerebellar disturbance which has a good prognosis.

4.12

(a)	FALSE	– It is commoner in middle aged and elderly.
(b)	FALSE	– It is confined to the segmental distribution of one or more spinal (or trigeminal) nerves. It is unilateral.
(c)	TRUE	
(d)	TRUE	
(e)	TRUE	– Particularly in the immunocompromised patient in whom the incidence is higher.

4.13

(a)	TRUE	– Gram-negative diplococcus.
(b)	TRUE	– Gram-negative bacillus.
(c)	FALSE	– Gram-positive coccus.
(d)	FALSE	– Gram-positive coccus.
(e)	FALSE	– This is a virus (picornavirus, RNA virus).

4.14

(a)	FALSE	– *Streptococcus pneumoniae* is the commonest organism in the elderly. *E. coli* meningitis is most common in neonates.
(b)	FALSE	– It is usually positive. This is the pain produced on extension of the knee with the hip flexed due to meningeal irritation of the lumbar nerves.
(c)	FALSE	– Chloramphenicol 2 g daily in the adult (50–100 mg/kg/day for children) is the drug of choice for 10 days.
(d)	TRUE	– It occurs in 50% of cases.
(e)	FALSE	– It is either very low (compared with blood sugar) or undetectable.

4.15

(a)	TRUE	– Occurs in 5% and is permanent involving one or both ears due to labyrinthitis.
(b)	FALSE	– This is a seventh nerve palsy (lower motor neurone) with an unknown aetiology. Cranial nerve palsies (III, IV, VI or VII) can occur and are transient.
(c)	TRUE	
(d)	FALSE	– Polyarthritis is rare but does not leave permanent joint damage.
(e)	TRUE	– Occurs months later and is usually focal.

4.16 **Meningicoccal meningitis:**
(a) Requires a 2 day course of penicillin for all contacts.
(b) May cause adrenal haemorrhage.
(c) Is treated with sulphonamides.
(d) Is associated with a negligible mortality.
(e) Is associated with a raised CSF protein.

4.17 **The following are characteristic of measles infection:**
(a) Koplik's spots occurring on the trunk.
(b) Conjunctivitis.
(c) An incubation period of 48 h.
(d) Absence of systemic upset.
(e) High infectivity by droplet spread.

4.18 **Regarding the complications of measles virus:**
(a) Pneumonia and bronchitis are the most common.
(b) They are more likely to occur in poor social conditions.
(c) Encephalitis is common.
(d) Appendicitis may occur.
(e) Subacute sclerosing panencephalitis may occur 1–4 days after the appearance of the rash.

4.19 **Viral meningitis:**
(a) Results in a very low CSF sugar concentration.
(b) Is more commonly caused by Influenza A.
(c) Is associated with a substantial mortality.
(d) Due to mumps virus is always accompanied by parotitis.
(e) Results in a lymphocytosis in the CSF.

4.20 **The following antibiotics can be used safely in pregnancy:**
(a) Gentamicin.
(b) Tetracycline.
(c) Ampicillin.
(d) Cotrimoxazole.
(e) Cephalexin.

4.16

(a)	FALSE	–	Rifampicin is the drug of choice. Contacts are often carriers of the organism.
(b)	TRUE	–	This is the rapidly fatal Waterhouse–Friederichsen syndrome which is caused by septicaemic shock and disseminated intravascular coagulation.
(c)	FALSE	–	10% of strains are resistant. High-dose intravenous benzyl-penicillin is used.
(d)	FALSE	–	Overall mortality is 5–10% with treatment (65% if untreated).
(e)	TRUE	–	2–5 g/l (normal = 0.2–0.5 g/l).

4.17

(a)	FALSE	–	These are off-white granules which occur in the buccal mucosa opposite the molars in 90% of cases. A maculo-papular rash occurs on the body.
(b)	TRUE	–	The eyes are commonly red and watery.
(c)	FALSE	–	This is 7–21 days (10 days on average).
(d)	FALSE	–	There is abrupt onset of fever, malaise and upper respiratory tract catarrh. The rash occurs on day 4 of the illness.
(e)	TRUE		

4.18

(a)	TRUE	–	These account for 4% of cases. Due to secondary bacterial infection.
(b)	TRUE		
(c)	FALSE	–	It is rare and there is no association between the severity of measles and the incidence of encephalitis.
(d)	TRUE		
(e)	FALSE	–	This is a rare, often fatal late complication occurring months to years after an attack of measles.

4.19

(a)	FALSE	–	CSF sugar is normal (approximately 1.7 mmol/l below blood sugar level), except in mumps meningitis when CSF sugar is extremely low.
(b)	FALSE	–	Coxsackie and ECHO viruses are commonest causes.
(c)	FALSE	–	Recovery is complete and there is no mortality.
(d)	FALSE	–	One-quarter to one-third of cases do not have parotitis.
(e)	TRUE		

4.20

(a)	FALSE	–	May cause auditory or vestibular nerve damage in second and third trimesters.
(b)	FALSE	–	Causes dental discolouration and maternal hepatotoxicity in second and third trimesters.
(c)	TRUE		
(d)	FALSE	–	Teratogenic if given in first trimester. May cause neonatal haemolysis and increased risk of kernicterus if given in third trimester.
(e)	TRUE		

4.21 **Rubella:**
(a) Causes a severe systemic upset.
(b) Causes enlargement of the posterior cervical lymph glands.
(c) Produces a rash which initially appears on the abdomen.
(d) Is more likely to cause teratogenic effects if acquired in the second trimester than the first.
(e) Vaccination should be given during pregnancy if the patient is not immune.

4.22 **Mumps may cause:**
(a) Pancreatitis.
(b) Infertility.
(c) Deafness.
(d) Encephalomyelitis.
(e) Swelling of the submandibular glands.

4.23 **Acute epiglottitis:**
(a) Is caused by parainfluenza virus.
(b) Responds to acyclovir.
(c) Is uncommon over 5 years of age.
(d) Requires hospitalization and nursing in a humid atmosphere.
(e) May cause airways obstruction.

4.24 **The following organisms can cause food poisoning:**
(a) *Staphylococcus aureus.*
(b) *Corynebacterium diphtheriae.*
(c) *Streptococcus viridans.*
(d) *Bacillus cereus.*
(e) *Clostridium perfringens.*

4.25 **Infective hepatitis:**
(a) Is caused by Hepatitis B virus.
(b) May be transmitted by contaminated water.
(c) Is commoner in summer months.
(d) May result in a carrier state.
(e) Is followed by lasting immunity.

4.21
(a)   FALSE   –   It is a mild illness and is often subclinical.
(b)   TRUE   –   This is characteristic.
(c)   FALSE   –   The macular rash usually begins on the face and neck and spreads within 24 h to the trunk and limbs.
(d)   FALSE   –   Percentage of cases suffering from fetal damage is 50% in the first trimester and 5% in the second.
(e)   FALSE   –   Vaccination is now recommended for all girls age 10–14 years. Pregnancy is a contraindication due to risk of teratogenicity.

4.22
(a)   TRUE
(b)   TRUE   –   This is rare and follows mumps orchitis which occurs in the post-pubertal patient.
(c)   TRUE
(d)   TRUE   –   Rare and often fatal.
(e)   TRUE

4.23
(a)   FALSE   –   This causes croup. *Haemophilus influenzae* causes epiglottitis.
(b)   FALSE   –   Chloramphenicol is the drug of choice.
(c)   TRUE
(d)   TRUE
(e)   TRUE

4.24
(a)   TRUE
(b)   FALSE
(c)   FALSE
(d)   TRUE
(e)   TRUE

4.25
(a)   FALSE   –   It is caused by Hepatitis A virus.
(b)   TRUE
(c)   FALSE   –   Peak incidence is in autumn and winter.
(d)   FALSE
(e)   TRUE

4.26 Hepatitis B:
(a) Is transmitted by blood products.
(b) Is usually transmitted transplacentally if the mother becomes infected.
(c) Results in carrier states of Hepatitis B surface antigen more commonly in Down's syndrome.
(d) Resulting in persistant Hepatitis E antigen carrier status is associated with greater infectivity than Hepatitis B surface antigen carrier states.
(e) Has an incubation period of 7 days.

4.27 Regarding viral hepatitis:
(a) Chronic active hepatitis may follow Hepatitis A infection.
(b) Hepatoma is associated with chronic hepatitis B surface antigen carrier states.
(c) There is usually a neutrophil leucocytosis.
(d) Hepatitis B vaccine affords protection.
(e) Splenomegaly may occur.

4.28 Rabies:
(a) May be transmitted by the vampire bat.
(b) Is endemic in the UK.
(c) In the human causes a personality change.
(d) Is usually fatal.
(e) Is caused by an organism which is a Gram-negative bacillus.

4.29 Erysipelas:
(a) Is a superficial infection of the skin.
(b) Is most common on the trunk.
(c) Is caused by group A streptococci.
(d) Responds to penicillin.
(e) Is commoner in children.

4.30 Regarding tetracycline antibiotics:
(a) They are used in the treatment of Q fever.
(b) They are effective in *Mycoplasma* pneumonia.
(c) They may cause renal failure.
(d) They are helpful in treating bronchitis caused by secondary bacterial infection in children following an attack of measles.
(e) Pseudomembranous colitis may occur as a complication.

4.26
(a) TRUE – Commonly seen in drug addicts sharing infected needles.
(b) FALSE – This is rare. Infants acquire it by transmission through the mucosa of eyes or gastrointestinal tract soon after birth.
(c) TRUE
(d) TRUE
(e) FALSE – It is 6 weeks to 6 months (average 100 days).

4.27
(a) FALSE – It sometimes is a sequel to Hepatitis B or Hepatitis non-A non-B infection.
(b) TRUE
(c) FALSE – There is a leucopenia and relative lymphocytosis.
(d) TRUE
(e) TRUE – This is uncommon but mild.

4.28
(a) TRUE – The bat is the only healthy carrier. Other carriers, i.e. dogs, foxes and cats, succumb to the disease.
(b) FALSE – It is usually imported from Europe.
(c) TRUE – The patient exhibits excitability, fear and anxiety.
(d) TRUE
(e) FALSE – Rabies is caused by rabies virus which is a rhabdovirus.

4.29
(a) FALSE – It is an infection of the skin and subcutaneous tissues with oedema and systemic upset.
(b) FALSE – The face (causing a 'butterfly' rash) and the lower limbs are the commonest sites.
(c) TRUE
(d) TRUE – Erythromycin is effective in the penicillin sensitive patient.
(e) FALSE – It is commoner in the adult (> 40 years of age).

4.30
(a) TRUE
(b) TRUE
(c) TRUE
(d) FALSE – They should never be used in children as they are deposited in growing bones and teeth causing staining and occasionally dental hypoplasia.
(e) TRUE – This can occur with almost any antibiotic.

4.31 **Regarding Lassa fever:**
(a) It is primarily transmitted by airborne infection.
(b) It is caused by a virus.
(c) It is transmitted by the sandfly.
(d) Full recovery is the rule.
(e) Haemorrhage may occur.

4.32 **The following are clinical features of poliomyelitis:**
(a) Peripheral neuropathy.
(b) Neurological signs are symmetrical.
(c) Flaccid paralysis involving the legs more than the arms.
(d) Dysphagia.
(e) Generalized maculopapular rash.

4.33 **Coxsackie virus infection is associated with:**
(a) Myocarditis.
(b) Peripheral neuropathy.
(c) Bornholms' disease.
(d) Lower motor neurone paralysis.
(e) Cholecystitis.

4.34 **Regarding neonatal meningitis:**
(a) *Niesseria meningitidis* is a common cause.
(b) Neck stiffness is a common clinical feature.
(c) *Escherichia coli* is a common cause.
(d) It is commoner in low birth weight infants.
(e) The mortality is high.

4.35 **Candidiasis:**
(a) Is more common in diabetics.
(b) May complicate treatment with antibiotics.
(c) Is usually treated with intravenous amphotericin B.
(d) May cause a vaginitis.
(e) Is usually accompanied by systemic upset.

4.31
(a)	FALSE	– It is transmitted by infected body fluids.
(b)	TRUE	
(c)	FALSE	– Rodents are the vectors.
(d)	FALSE	– In Europeans the mortality is 50%. The disease is milder in Africa where it is endemic.
(e)	TRUE	

4.32
(a)	FALSE	– Sensory changes do not occur. The virus destroys anterior horn cells in the spinal cord.
(b)	FALSE	
(c)	TRUE	
(d)	TRUE	– Due to involvement of lower brain stem nuclei causing a bulbar palsy.
(e)	FALSE	

4.33
(a)	TRUE	
(b)	FALSE	
(c)	TRUE	– This is epidemic myalgia caused by group B viruses.
(d)	TRUE	– It may be indistinguishable from poliomyelitis.
(e)	FALSE	

4.34
(a)	FALSE	
(b)	FALSE	– The classical signs are often lacking. The baby is irritable and vomiting. A bulging fontanelle may be present.
(c)	TRUE	
(d)	TRUE	
(e)	TRUE	

4.35
(a)	TRUE	
(b)	TRUE	
(c)	FALSE	– Is used for severe infections usually in the immuno-compromised. It is a toxic drug and may cause anaemia and renal failure.
(d)	TRUE	
(e)	FALSE	

4.36 **Whooping cough:**
(a) Is commonly caused by *Bordetella parapertussis*.
(b) Is usually a recurrent illness.
(c) May be complicated by bronchiectasis.
(d) May be complicated by convulsions.
(e) Is treated with tetracycline.

4.37 **Whooping cough vaccine:**
(a) May cause brain damage.
(b) Is given at age 2 years.
(c) Should be avoided if there is a family history of asthma.
(d) Is not recommended in a child with cerebral palsy.
(e) Is given with the measles and BCG vaccine.

4.38 **Erythema nodosum may be caused by infections with the following organisms:**
(a) *Mycobacterium tuberculosus*.
(b) *Streptococcus pyogenes*.
(c) Q fever.
(d) Respiratory syncytial virus.
(e) Rhinovirus.

4.39 **Toxic shock syndrome:**
(a) May result in desquamation.
(b) Is caused by a streptococcal infection.
(c) Is treated with intravenous benzylpenicillin.
(d) Is associated with vaginal infection.
(e) May result in thrombocytopenia.

4.40 **The following are common clinical features of typhoid fever:**
(a) Diarrhoea.
(b) Splenomegaly.
(c) Bronchopneumonia.
(d) Convulsions.
(e) Dysphagia.

4.36

(a)	FALSE	– *Bordetella pertussis* is the most common infecting organism. Infection with *B. parapertussis* is rare.
(b)	FALSE	– Second attacks of whooping cough are rare.
(c)	TRUE	
(d)	TRUE	– Usually febrile convulsions but may follow a cyanotic episode when they are due to anoxia.
(e)	FALSE	– *B. pertussis* is sensitive to erythromycin and tetracycline. The latter should never be used in children. Antibiotics do not seem to affect the progression of whooping cough.

4.37

(a)	TRUE	– This is very rare. The risk of permanent brain damage is 1 in 310 000 injections.
(b)	FALSE	– The mortality is highest under 2 years and the vaccine is given with the 'triple vaccine' at 3 months, 6 months and 1 year.
(c)	FALSE	
(d)	TRUE	– It should be avoided in children who suffer from convulsions or have a neurological disorder.
(e)	FALSE	– This 'triple vaccine' is against whooping cough, diphtheria and tetanus and is given with oral polio vaccine.

4.38

(a)	TRUE	
(b)	TRUE	
(c)	TRUE	
(d)	FALSE	– This causes bronchiolitis in babies.
(e)	FALSE	

4.39

(a)	TRUE	
(b)	FALSE	– It is caused by a staphylococcal toxin, (pyrogenic exotoxin A).
(c)	FALSE	– Flucloxacillin is the antibiotic of choice.
(d)	TRUE	– It is related to menstruation and tampon usage.
(e)	TRUE	

4.40

(a)	TRUE	– 50% of cases develop diarrhoea in the second week.
(b)	TRUE	
(c)	TRUE	– This may occur, usually in second week.
(d)	FALSE	– Delirium, formerly called the 'typhoid state' may occur in the third week of the illness but convulsions are rare.
(e)	FALSE	

4.41 **Regarding syphilis:**
(a) 'Snail track' ulcers occur in primary syphilis.
(b) The chancre is a feature of primary syphilis.
(c) Tertiary syphilis takes 2 weeks to develop.
(d) Erythromycin is the first drug of choice.
(e) The Wasserman Reaction (WR) is 100% specific for syphilis.

4.42 **Gonorrhoea:**
(a) Is due to a Gram-negative diplococcus.
(b) May be asymptomatic in the female.
(c) Usually presents as epididymo-orchitis in the male.
(d) Is treated with penicillin.
(e) May lead to sterility.

4.43 **Regarding typhoid fever:**
(a) Chronic carrier states are most likely to occur if antibiotics are used.
(b) Blood cultures are usually negative.
(c) May be complicated by cholecystitis.
(d) May be complicated by intestinal perforation.
(e) It is a milder disease than paratyphoid fever.

4.44 **The following are recognized clinical features of toxoplasmosis:**
(a) Lymphadenopathy.
(b) Shock.
(c) Uveitis.
(d) Flaccid paralysis.
(e) Hepatitis.

4.45 **Malaria:**
(a) Is endemic in the UK.
(b) Is transmitted by the male mosquito.
(c) Is a mild disease if caused by *Plasmodium falciparum*.
(d) Often causes splenomegaly.
(e) May lead to nephrotic syndrome.

4.41

(a) FALSE – These are found on the mucosal membranes of the genitalia and mouth and are a feature of secondary syphilis.

(b) TRUE – This is a pink macule which becomes papular and ulcerates.

(c) FALSE – This usually takes 10 or more years.

(d) FALSE – Procaine penicillin is used and for those who are sensitive to penicillin tetracycline is used.

(e) FALSE – It may give false positives with glandular fever and SLE and other generalized diseases.

4.42

(a) TRUE – *Neisseria gonorrhoea.*

(b) TRUE – 50% of females have no symptoms.

(c) FALSE – Usually there is an anterior urethritis causing dysuria and a discharge.

(d) TRUE

(e) TRUE – Infection may spread to the pelvis (pelvic inflammatory disease) and result in sterility.

4.43

(a) FALSE – Chloramphenicol is the drug of choice in all proven cases. It does not affect the carrier state.

(b) FALSE – Usually positive in the first two weeks.

(c) TRUE – This is common, usually subclinical and is an important factor in subsequent faecal carriage.

(d) TRUE

(e) FALSE

4.44

(a) TRUE

(b) FALSE

(c) TRUE

(d) FALSE

(e) TRUE

4.45

(a) FALSE – It is endemic in Asia, Africa, the Middle East and South and Central America.

(b) FALSE – It is transmitted by the female mosquito.

(c) FALSE – This is a severe form which may be fatal.

(d) TRUE

(e) TRUE – Usually chronic *Plasmodium malariae* infection.

4.46   Hydatid cysts:
(a)   Are caused by a bacterial infection.
(b)   Are more common in sheep-rearing countries.
(c)   May be asymptomatic.
(d)   Are usually subcutaneous.
(e)   Are uncommon in males.

4.47   Gas gangrene:
(a)   Is caused by *Clostridium botulinum*.
(b)   May occur after an amputation.
(c)   Is treated with intravenous tetracycline.
(d)   Requires surgical excision.
(e)   Is associated with a negligible mortality.

4.48   Metronidazole:
(a)   Is used in the treatment of toxoplasmosis.
(b)   Is used to treat giardiasis.
(c)   May cause a peripheral neuropathy.
(d)   Is poorly absorbed if taken orally.
(e)   Is effective against anaerobic bacteria.

4.49   Staphylococcal food poisoning:
(a)   Is caused by a toxin.
(b)   Has an average incubation period of 7 days.
(c)   Is treated with flucloxacillin.
(d)   May cause intestinal perforation.
(e)   Is caused by *Staphylococcus epidermidis*.

4.50   Salmonellosis:
(a)   Is most commonly caused by *Salmonella typhimurium*.
(b)   Resulting from infected food, can be recognized as the food has an altered taste.
(c)   May result in a severe colitis.
(d)   Is treated with chloramphenicol.
(e)   Is a notifiable disease.

4.46

(a)	FALSE	– *Echinococcus granulosus* is a small tapeworm causing the cyst.
(b)	TRUE	– As sheep are the usual intermediate host.
(c)	TRUE	
(d)	FALSE	– Most commonly occur in liver and lung.
(e)	FALSE	

4.47

(a)	FALSE	– Usually the anaerobes *Cl. perfringens*, *Cl. septicum* and *Cl. oedematiens*.
(b)	TRUE	– Ischaemic areas which are wounded are at risk.
(c)	FALSE	– Penicillin is the drug of choice. Metronidazole is equally effective.
(d)	TRUE	– Hyperbaric oxygen may reduce spread and limit excision.
(e)	FALSE	

4.48

(a)	FALSE	
(b)	TRUE	
(c)	TRUE	
(d)	FALSE	– It is well absorbed and can given serum levels equal to when given intravenously. The intravenous form is expensive and should be prescribed selectively.
(e)	TRUE	

4.49

(a)	TRUE	
(b)	FALSE	– The toxin is preformed in the food and hence the incubation period is 2–4 hours.
(c)	FALSE	– Treatment is sympathetic and the illness short-lived (24–48 h).
(d)	FALSE	
(e)	FALSE	– *Staphylococcus aureus* is the pathogen.

4.50

(a)	TRUE	
(b)	FALSE	
(c)	TRUE	
(d)	FALSE	– Antibiotics do not influence the course of the disease. However, they are used in the presence of septicaemia.
(e)	TRUE	

4.51 **The following are associated with bloody diarrhoea:**
(a) Dysentery.
(b) Campylobacteriosis.
(c) Staphylococcal enteritis.
(d) Salmonellosis.
(e) Brucellosis.

4.52 **Brucellosis:**
(a) May be transmitted by pasteurized milk.
(b) Has an incubation period of 24 h.
(c) Is associated with fever.
(d) May cause spontaneous abortion in humans.
(e) Is treated with tetracycline.

4.53 **Regarding bacillary dysentry:**
(a) It is endemic in the UK.
(b) Chronic carrier states are common.
(c) It is caused by *Entamoeba histolytica*.
(d) It is associated with a high mortality.
(e) It is transmitted by faeces of an infected case.

4.54 **The following are features of infection with *Campylobacter jejuni*:**
(a) Myalagia.
(b) Colicky abdominal pain.
(c) Vesicular rash.
(d) Uveitis.
(e) Arthritis.

4.55 **Giardiasis:**
(a) Is caused by a virus.
(b) Causes fat malabsorption.
(c) Is treated with ampicillin.
(d) Has been eradicated by vaccination programmes in the UK.
(e) Is commoner in children.

4.51
(a) TRUE
(b) TRUE
(c) FALSE
(d) TRUE
(e) FALSE – This does not produce a gasteroenteritis.

4.52
(a) FALSE – *Brucella* species are killed by pasteurization and can be transmitted by unpasteurized milk or cheese.
(b) FALSE – It is usually 2–4 weeks.
(c) TRUE
(d) FALSE – *Brucella abortus* causes spontaneous abortion in cattle.
(e) TRUE – Streptomycin is given with tetracycline for 3 weeks followed by tetracycline alone for another 3 weeks.

4.53
(a) TRUE – There is an increased incidence in winter.
(b) FALSE – It is rare.
(c) FALSE – This causes amoebic dysentery. Bacillary dysentery is caused by the *Shigella* group of organisms.
(d) FALSE – Only 1–2 deaths per year usually in those with pre-existing disease and the elderly.
(e) TRUE

4.54
(a) TRUE
(b) TRUE
(c) FALSE – Erythema nodosum may occur.
(d) FALSE
(e) TRUE – A reactive arthritis may occur particularly in individuals with HLA B27.

4.55
(a) FALSE – It is caused by a flagellated protozoa, *Giardia intestinalis*.
(b) TRUE
(c) FALSE – Metronidazole is the drug of choice.
(d) FALSE
(e) TRUE

4.56 Pseudomembranous colitis:
(a) Is due to *Clostridium difficile* infection.
(b) May follow treatment with ampicillin.
(c) Is associated with a leucopenia.
(d) Causes yellow-white plaques which are seen on sigmoidoscopy.
(e) Is treated with clindamycin.

4.57 Acquired immune deficiency syndrome (AIDS):
(a) May present with *Pneumocystis carinii* pneumonia.
(b) Is transmitted by airborne infection.
(c) Is associated with Kaposi's sarcoma.
(d) Is rare in homosexuals.
(e) Is caused by bacterial infection.

4.58 Tetanus:
(a) Is a notifiable disease.
(b) Is uncommon now due to a vaccination programme.
(c) Is associated with no mortality.
(d) Produces lifelong immunity on recovery from an attack.
(e) Is commoner in the elderly.

4.59 Regarding leptospirosis:
(a) It is transmitted to humans from infected animals.
(b) When due to *Leptospira icterohaemorrhagiae* is a mild influenza-like illness.
(c) Acute renal failure may occur.
(d) Conjunctival haemorrhage may be present.
(e) A vaccine is available for humans.

4.60 Erythromycin:
(a) Is used to treat Legionnaire's disease.
(b) Is useful as a second choice antibiotic in the penicillin sensitive patient.
(c) Is only available in oral form.
(d) Commonly causes nausea.
(e) Is used to treat *Mycoplasma* pneumonia.

4.56
(a) TRUE – Gram-positive anaerobic bacillus.
(b) TRUE – Almost any antibiotic may cause it.
(c) FALSE – There is usually a leucocytosis.
(d) TRUE
(e) FALSE – This is a common cause of the colitis. It is treated with vancomycin or metronidazole.

4.57
(a) TRUE
(b) FALSE – It is transmitted by blood and its products (semen).
(c) TRUE – This is a purple skin lesion.
(d) FALSE – It is most common in homosexuals and intravenous drug abusers.
(e) FALSE – It is caused by a virus.

4.58
(a) FALSE
(b) TRUE
(c) FALSE – Mortality in untreated cases is 60% and 10–20% when treated.
(d) FALSE – Second attacks can occur and survivors require active immunization.
(e) TRUE – There are about 50 cases a year in England and Wales.

4.59
(a) TRUE – From urine of infected animals, e.g. rats.
(b) FALSE – Milder forms are with *L. canicola* and *L. hebdomadis* infection.
(c) TRUE
(d) TRUE
(e) FALSE – Dogs can be vaccinated against *L. canicola* infection.

4.60
(a) TRUE
(b) TRUE – It has a similar spectrum to penicillin.
(c) FALSE
(d) TRUE
(e) TRUE

5 Haematology

5.1 **The following may cause a normochromic, normocytic anaemia:**
(a) B_{12} deficiency.
(b) Rheumatoid arthritis.
(c) Menorrhagia.
(d) Hypothyroidism.
(e) Folate deficiency.

5.2 **Regarding iron deficiency anaemia treated with oral iron therapy:**
(a) The haemoglobin rises by 0.1 g/dl each week.
(b) Constipation is a common side-effect.
(c) Treatment is discontinued when the haemoglobin returns to normal.
(d) Ferrous fumarate is the iron salt of first choice in replacement therapy.
(e) If due to Crohn's disease treatment will be effective.

5.3 **Erythropoiesis:**
(a) Occurs in the bone marrow throughout fetal life.
(b) Results in the production of normoblasts which are nucleated red cells normally seen in the peripheral blood.
(c) Is stimulated by the hormone erythropoietin.
(d) Results in red cells which contain a nucleus.
(e) Requires iron.

5.4 **The normal red cell:**
(a) Has a lifespan of 120 days.
(b) Contains haemoglobin.
(c) Is destroyed in the kidneys.
(d) Is a rigid structure.
(e) Has a volume of 1 millilitre.

5.5 **The following cause a macrocytosis (large red cell, MCV > 100 fl):**
(a) Alcoholism.
(b) Hypothyroidism.
(c) Chronic renal failure.
(d) Sideroblastic anaemia.
(e) Haemolysis.

5.1

(a)	FALSE	–	This produces a macrocytic normochromic anaemia.
(b)	TRUE		
(c)	FALSE	–	This produces a microcytic hypochromic anaemia (iron deficiency anaemia).
(d)	TRUE		
(e)	FALSE	–	See (a).

5.2

(a)	FALSE	–	Haemoglobin should rise by 1 g/dl each week providing there is no continued blood loss or malabsorption.
(b)	TRUE		
(c)	FALSE	–	Treatment should be continued for 3 months after haemoglobin returns to normal to replenish body iron stores.
(d)	FALSE	–	Ferrous sulphate is the cheapest salt and is the first choice.
(e)	FALSE	–	If the anaemia is due to malabsorption then iron should be given parenterally (intramuscular).

5.3

(a)	FALSE	–	Haemopoeisis occurs in the fetal liver and spleen until 7 months. After this the bone marrow is the site where this occurs.
(b)	FALSE	–	Normoblasts are nucleated cells in the red cell production line but are not normally seen in the peripheral blood.
(c)	TRUE		
(d)	FALSE	–	Red cells are non-nucleated biconcave discs.
(e)	TRUE		

5.4

(a)	TRUE		
(b)	TRUE	–	This is the molecule which carries oxygen to tissues and CO_2 from them.
(c)	FALSE	–	Red cell destruction occurs in the reticuloendothelial system (bone marrow, liver, spleen).
(d)	FALSE	–	It is flexible as it is 8 μm in diameter and it has to travel through the microcirculation whose minimum diameter is 3.5 μm.
(e)	FALSE	–	The mean red cell volume (MCV) is 80–95 femtolitres.

5.5

(a)	TRUE		
(b)	TRUE		
(c)	FALSE	–	This causes a normochromic normocytic anaemia.
(d)	TRUE		
(e)	TRUE	–	Due to large numbers of reticulocytes (which are larger than mature red cells) because of increased turnover of cells.

5.6 **Heparin:**
(a) May be given orally.
(b) Inhibits clotting.
(c) May have its effects reversed by protamine.
(d) Has a half-life of 24 h
(e) May cause alopecia.

5.7 **Regarding iron absorption:**
(a) It is increased in preganancy.
(b) It occurs predominantly in the terminal ileum.
(c) It is enhanced by acidic conditions.
(d) It is enhanced by desferrioxamine.
(e) After absorption it exists as free iron in the ferrous form in peripheral blood.

5.8 **The following are recognized clinical features of iron deficiency anaemia:**
(a) Finger clubbing.
(b) Glossitis.
(c) Jaundice.
(d) Dysphagia.
(e) Conjunctivitis.

5.9 **Iron deficiency anaemia:**
(a) May be caused by menorrhagia.
(b) Results in a reticulocytosis.
(c) Is associated with spherical red cells.
(d) May be the presenting feature of a caecal carcinoma.
(e) Is associated with a leucopenia.

5.10 **Regarding sideroblastic anaemia:**
(a) The ring sideroblast is seen in the peripheral blood.
(b) Bone marrow iron stores are depleted.
(c) It may respond to pyridoxine.
(d) It may be caused by isoniazid.
(e) The red cells are normochromic.

5.6

(a) FALSE – It is not absorbed from the gastrointestinal tract and therefore must be given parenterally.

(b) TRUE – It inhibits almost every sequence in the clotting mechanism in particular thromboplastin and thrombin generation.

(c) TRUE

(d) FALSE – The average half life is 60–80 min.

(e) TRUE – Other common side-effects are paraesthesiae, thrombocytopenia, urticaria and osteoporosis (with prolonged use).

5.7

(a) TRUE – Normally 5–10% of dietary iron is absorbed. This increases to 20–30% in pregnancy.

(b) FALSE – Mainly through duodenum but also through jejunum.

(c) TRUE – Vitamin C for example enhances absorption.

(d) FALSE – This is an iron chelating agent.

(e) FALSE – Iron is bound to transferrin in the ferric form in blood. There is normally no free iron in blood.

5.8

(a) FALSE – Spoon-shaped nails (koilonychia) may occur.

(b) TRUE

(c) FALSE

(d) TRUE – Due to formation of a pharyngeal web (Paterson–Kelly or Plummer–Vinson syndrome).

(e) FALSE

5.9

(a) TRUE

(b) FALSE – The reticulocyte count is low (normal 0.5–2%) but increases with treatment.

(c) FALSE

(d) TRUE

(e) FALSE

5.10

(a) FALSE – These are abnormal erythroblasts containing iron granules which are arranged in a ring around the nucleus. They are seen in the bone marrow.

(b) FALSE – It is due to a defect of haem synthesis and iron stores are normal.

(c) TRUE

(d) TRUE – Isoniazid is a B_6 antagonist.

(e) FALSE – They are hypochromic. They are microcytic also in the hereditary form but are sometimes macrocytic in the acquired form.

5.11 **Warfarin:**
(a) Has a half-life of 4 h.
(b) Inhibits the synthesis of vitamin K dependent clotting factors.
(c) Is metabolized by the kidney.
(d) Is used to dissolve thrombi, i.e. produce thrombolysis.
(e) Interacts with alcohol.

5.12 **The following drugs may cause a neutropenia:**
(a) Carbimazole.
(b) Cyclophosphamide.
(c) Atenolol.
(d) Glibenclamide.
(e) Phenytoin.

5.13 **The following are clinical features of multiple myeloma:**
(a) Bone pain.
(b) Hypocalcaemia.
(c) Polycythaemia.
(d) Renal failure.
(e) Bleeding tendency.

5.14 **Regarding multiple myeloma:**
(a) The commonest serum paraprotein is IgG.
(b) Bence Jones protein may occur in the urine in the absence of a serum paraprotein.
(c) Renal impairment is a good prognostic sign.
(d) Amyloidosis may occur.
(e) The ESR is less than 30 mm/h.

5.15 **The following are causes of a leucoerythroblastic anaemia:**
(a) Severe haemorrhage.
(b) Multiple myeloma.
(c) Chronic lymphocytic leukaemia.
(d) Acute myeloid leukaemia.
(e) Megaloblastic anaemia.

5.11
(a) FALSE – Half-life is about 44 h.
(b) TRUE – These are factors II, VII, IX and X.
(c) FALSE – It is metabolized by the liver.
(d) FALSE – It prevents further thrombus formation but is not a thrombolytic agent.
(e) TRUE – Alcohol enhances the effect of warfarin. Many drugs also interact with warfarin.

5.12
(a) TRUE – Patients should be warned if they develop any infection, e.g. sore throat, to visit the doctor.
(b) TRUE – All cytotoxics may cause aplastic anaemia (decreased red blood cells, decreased white blood cells, decreased platelets).
(c) FALSE
(d) TRUE
(e) TRUE – May cause an aplastic anaemia. Also causes a megloblastic anaemia due to the inhibition of folate absorption.

5.13
(a) TRUE – Pathological fractures may occur.
(b) FALSE – Hypercalcaemia occurs resulting in polydipsia, polyuria, constipation and mental disturbance.
(c) FALSE – Anaemia is usual.
(d) TRUE
(e) TRUE – Myeloma protein interferes with platelet function and coagulation factors. Thrombocytopenia occurs in advanced disease.

5.14
(a) TRUE – IgG in two-thirds of cases and IgA in one-third. IgM and IgD paraproteinaemia are rare.
(b) TRUE – This occurs in 15% of cases.
(c) FALSE – If the blood urea is > 14 mmol/l at presentation the median survival is only a few months.
(d) TRUE
(e) FALSE – It is usually very high.

5.15
(a) TRUE
(b) TRUE
(c) FALSE
(d) TRUE
(e) TRUE – Erythroblasts and primitive white cells are found in the peripheral blood. It is due to extramedullary haemopoeisis or infiltration of the marrow.

5.16 **The following are causes of a raised platelet count (thrombocythaemia):**
(a) Malignancy.
(b) Rheumatoid arthritis.
(c) B_{12}deficiency.
(d) Chloramphenicol.
(e) Gold salts.

5.17 **The following are caues of a lymphocytosis ($> 3.5 \times 10^9$/l):**
(a) Pneumococcal pneumonia.
(b) Chronic lymphocytic leukaemia.
(c) Infectious mononucleosis.
(d) Hay fever.
(e) Meningococcal meningitis.

5.18 **Regarding Waldenstrom's macroglobulinaemia:**
(a) It is commoner in women.
(b) An IgG paraproteinaemia occurs.
(c) Results in a hyperviscosity syndrome.
(d) Hepatosplenomegaly may occur.
(e) Retinal haemorrhages may occur.

5.19 **The following are features of megaloblastic anaemia:**
(a) Jaundice.
(b) Purpura.
(c) Malar flush.
(d) Angular stomatitis.
(e) Neutrophils with hypersegmented nuclei.

5.20 **Regarding vitamin B_{12}:**
(a) It is found mainly in vegetables.
(b) It is absorbed through the duodenum.
(c) It requires intrinsic factor produced by the gastric parietal cells for its absorption.
(d) Deficiency may occur due to increased utilization in pregnancy.
(e) Body stores are sufficient for 3 months.

5.16
(a) TRUE
(b) TRUE
(c) FALSE – The platelet count is usually low.
(d) FALSE – May cause an aplastic anaemia.
(e) FALSE – May cause an aplastic anaemia.

5.17
(a) FALSE – Bacterial infection result in a neutrophil leucocytosis.
(b) TRUE
(c) TRUE
(d) FALSE – Produces an eosinophilia.
(e) FALSE – see (a).

5.18
(a) FALSE – Commoner in men over 50 years of age.
(b) FALSE – There is a proliferation of cells which produce an IgM
                    paraprotein.
(c) TRUE   – This causes visual disturbances, confusion, lethargy,
                    muscle weakness, nervous system symptoms and signs
                    of congestive heart failure.
(d) TRUE   – Frequently seen.
(e) TRUE   – Also engorged veins, exudates and blurred disc.

5.19
(a) TRUE   – Usually mild due to increased ineffective erythropoiesis,
                    increased breakdown of haemoglobin and shortened red
                    cell survival.
(b) TRUE   – Due to thrombocytopenia.
(c) FALSE
(d) TRUE
(e) TRUE

5.20
(a) FALSE – Its origin is liver, fish and dairy produce.
(b) FALSE – It is absorbed through the terminal ileum.
(c) TRUE
(d) FALSE – There is no syndrome of deficiency due to increased
                    utilization or loss of vitamin B_{12}.
(e) FALSE – Body stores (mainly liver) are sufficent for 2–4 years.
                    They are used at 1–2 μg/day.

5.21 Pernicious anaemia (PA):
(a) Is commoner in women.
(b) Is associated with blood group AB.
(c) Is associated with intrinsic factor antibodies in the serum.
(d) May produce increased skin pigmentation.
(e) Is associated with premature greying of the hair.

5.22 The following are causes of folate deficiency:
(a) Pregnancy.
(b) Congestive heart failure.
(c) Malignancy.
(d) Psoriasis.
(e) Terminal ileal resection.

5.23 Regarding polycythaemia rubra vera:
(a) The total red cell volume is decreased.
(b) It is commoner in women.
(c) Pruritus may occur.
(d) Headaches may occur.
(e) Splenomegaly is a common finding.

5.24 The following are causes of polycythaemia:
(a) Cerebellar haemangioblastoma.
(b) Hepatoma.
(c) Renal carcinoma.
(d) Excess dietary iron.
(e) Crohn's disease.

5.25 The following are laboratory features of haemolytic anaemia:
(a) Reticulocytosis.
(b) Increased ESR.
(c) Microcytosis.
(d) Hyperbilirubinaemia.
(e) Increased serum haptoglobulins.

5.21

(a)	TRUE	– Ratio F : M is 1.6 : 1.
(b)	FALSE	– It is associated with blood group A.
(c)	TRUE	– Specific for PA and occurs in 50% of cases. Parietal cell antibody is less specific but occurs in 90% of the cases.
(d)	TRUE	– This is uncommon and reversible. Vitiligo may occur and is irreversible.
(e)	TRUE	

5.22

(a)	TRUE	– All pregnant women require supplements because of increased cell turnover. Supplementation before and in early pregnancy specifically reduces the incidence of neural tube defects.
(b)	TRUE	– Due to excess urinary folate loss.
(c)	TRUE	– Due to increased utilization in cell formation.
(d)	TRUE	
(e)	FALSE	– It is absorbed through duodenum and jejunum.

5.23

(a)	FALSE	– It is increased (> 36 ml/kg in men and > 32 ml/kg in women).
(b)	FALSE	– Sex incidence is equal.
(c)	TRUE	– Especially after a hot bath.
(d)	TRUE	– Due to the hyperviscosity syndrome it produces.
(e)	TRUE	– Occurs in two-thirds of patients.

5.24

(a)	TRUE	– Due to an inappropriate increase in erythropoietin.
(b)	TRUE	– Due to an inappropriate increase in erythropoietin.
(c)	TRUE	– Due to an inappropriate increase in erythropoietin.
(d)	FALSE	
(e)	FALSE	

5.25

(a)	TRUE	– Due to increased red cell production. The adult marrow is able to produce red cells at 6–8 times its normal rate.
(b)	FALSE	
(c)	FALSE	– Red cells are usually large.
(d)	TRUE	
(e)	FALSE	– Haptoglobins (haemoglobin binding protein) are reduced because the haemoglobin–haptoglobin complex is removed by reticuloendothelial cells.

5.26 **Regarding hereditary spherocytosis:**
(a) Surface area to volume ratio of red cells is increased.
(b) It has a sex-linked recessive inheritance pattern.
(c) Splenomegaly is a common finding.
(d) It is the commonest hereditary haemolytic anaemia in northern Europeans.
(e) The marrow produces red cells which are spherical.

5.27 **Regarding glucose 6-phosphate dehydrogenase deficiency:**
(a) Its inheritance is sex-linked.
(b) Blood count is normal between crises.
(c) Effects are most severe in Negroes.
(d) Haemolytic anaemia may be precipitated by diabetic keto-acidosis.
(e) Direct Coomb's test is positive.

5.28 **Sickle cell anaemia:**
(a) Is due to reduced synthesis of the B globin chain.
(b) Results in crises when exposed to low oxygen tensions.
(c) May be associated with leg ulcers.
(d) Is common in Scandinavians.
(e) Affords protection gainst *Plasmodium falciparium*, if subject has sickle cell trait.

5.29 **β-thalassaemia major:**
(a) Is due to reduced or absent production of the β globin chain.
(b) Results in hepatosplenomegaly.
(c) Is associated with a normochromic normocytic anaemia.
(d) Is treated with regular oral desferrioxamine.
(e) May be detected antenatally.

5.30 **Regarding autoimmune haemolytic anaemia 'warm' type:**
(a) IgM is the most common antibody on the red cells.
(b) The direct Coomb's test is negative.
(c) It may occur in association with *Mycoplasma* pneumonia.
(d) It may occur in association with chronic lymphocytic leukaemia.
(e) Steroids are used in its treatment.

5.26
(a)   FALSE – This is decreased.
(b)   FALSE – It is an autosomal dominant condition with variable expression.
(c)   TRUE   – Splenectomy is the treatment of choice but should be avoided in children because of the risk of pneumococcal infection. Pneumococcal vaccination is given before surgery.
(d)   TRUE
(e)   FALSE – The marrow produces normal biconcave red cells but they lose membrane as they circulate through the spleen and the rest of the reticuloendothelial system and the cell becomes spherical.

5.27
(a)   TRUE   – Affects males and carried by females.
(b)   TRUE
(c)   FALSE – Most severe in Mediterraneans, less severe in Orientals and usually mild in Negroes.
(d)   TRUE   – Also precipitated by acute infections, drugs, e.g. paracetamol, penicillin, and the fava bean.
(e)   FALSE

5.28
(a)   FALSE – It is due to a substitution of valine for glutamic acid in position 6 in the β chain.
(b)   TRUE   – Hb S is insoluble and forms crystals at low O_2 tensions. The red cells sickle.
(c)   TRUE   – Due to local ischaemia and vascular stasis.
(d)   FALSE – Mainly in tropical and subtropical areas.
(e)   TRUE   – This explains persistence of sickle cell trait (heterozygous form) in which 25–45% of haemoglobin is Hb S.

5.29
(a)   TRUE
(b)   TRUE   – Due to excessive red cell destruction, extramedullary haemopoiesis and iron overload. Expansion of bones occurs (frontal bossing) due to marrow hyperplasia.
(c)   FALSE – Severe hypochromic microcytic anaemia.
(d)   FALSE – Treated with regular transfusions. Desferrioxamine is given subcutaneously and chelates iron to prevent iron overload. This has improved the prognosis.
(e)   TRUE

5.30
(a)   FALSE – IgG is the most common in the 'warm' type and IgM in the 'cold' type.
(b)   FALSE
(c)   FALSE – This produces a 'cold' type autoimmune haemolytic anaemia.
(d)   TRUE
(e)   TRUE   – Splenectomy may also be useful. The offending cause (e.g. methyldopa) should also be treated or removed.

5.31 Aplastic anaemia:
(a) May be inherited as a Mendelian dominant condition.
(b) Is associated with recurrent infections.
(c) Produces hepatosplenomegaly.
(d) Causes a hypocellular bone marrow.
(e) Is treated with methotrexate.

5.32 The following may cause a monocytosis (count $> 0.8 \times 10^9/l$):
(a) Brucellosis.
(b) Hodgkin's disease.
(c) Glandular fever.
(d) Thyrotoxicosis.
(e) Toxoplasmosis.

5.33 Regarding immunoglobulins:
(a) They are a group of proteins produced by T lymphocytes.
(b) IgG is the most common.
(c) IgG is produced first in response to an antigen.
(d) Bence Jones protein consists of the heavy chains.
(e) IgG can travel across the placenta.

5.34 Disseminated intravascular coagulation (DIC):
(a) May occur secondary to septicaemmia.
(b) Is associated with an increased platelet count.
(c) Is associated with a haemolytic anaemia.
(d) Causes a decreased prothrombin time.
(e) Results in an increase in fibrinogen degradation products.

5.35 The following are aetiological factors in leukaemia/lymphoma:
(a) Epstein–Barr virus.
(b) Hereditary factors.
(c) Smoking.
(d) Chlorambucil.
(e) Ultraviolet light.

5.31
(a) FALSE – Fanconi type is a recessive disorder.
(b) TRUE – Due to neutropenia.
(c) FALSE
(d) TRUE
(e) FALSE – This is a cytotoxic drug which can cause aplastic anaemia.

5.32
(a) TRUE – Chronic bacterial infections, e.g. endocarditis, tuberculosis, can cause this.
(b) TRUE
(c) TRUE
(d) FALSE – Causes a lymphocytosis.
(e) FALSE – Causes a lymphocytosis.

5.33
(a) FALSE – They are produced by plasma cells and B lymphocytes.
(b) TRUE – Accounts for 80%.
(c) FALSE – IgM is produced first; IgG is produced subsequently and for a more prolonged period.
(d) FALSE – Light chains (either kappa or lambda).
(e) TRUE – IgM and IgA do not.

5.34
(a) TRUE – Usually Gram-negative.
(b) FALSE – These are low and contributes to the bleeding tendency.
(c) TRUE – Due to fragmentation of red cells as they pass through fibrin strands in small vessels.
(d) FALSE – It is increased.
(e) TRUE – In serum and urine. Serum fibrinogen is decreased.

5.35
(a) TRUE – Implicated in the aetiology of Burkitt's lymphoma.
(b) TRUE
(c) FALSE – This has not been proven.
(d) TRUE
(e) FALSE

5.36 **Regarding acute leukaemia:**
(a) This is more common than chronic leukaemia.
(b) Acute lymphoblastic leukaemia is the commonst leukaemia in adults.
(c) There is a proliferation of blast cells in the bone marrow.
(d) Acute myeloid leukaemia is associated with a proliferation of lymphoblasts in the bone marrow.
(e) Chromosome abnormalities are uncommon.

5.37 **The following are clinical features of acute leukaemia:**
(a) Skin pigmentation.
(b) Purpura.
(c) Rigors.
(d) Hepatosplenomegaly.
(e) Campbell de Morgan spots.

5.38 **Management of acute leukaemia may include:**
(a) A single cytotoxic agent.
(b) Splenectomy.
(c) Platelet concentrates to treat septicaemia.
(d) Radiation.
(e) Bone marrow transplantation.

5.39 **Regarding acute lymphoblastic leukaemia (ALL):**
(a) If it occurs in adult life the prognosis is good.
(b) The prognosis is worse in males.
(c) Meningeal involvement is common.
(d) Null-ALL is the commonest type.
(e) Lymphadenopathy is uncommon.

5.40 **Regarding acute myeloid leukaemia (AML):**
(a) The prognosis is better than in ALL with treatment.
(b) Promyelocytes may be seen in the peripheral blood.
(c) It is commoner in adults.
(d) Thrombocythaemia occurs.
(e) It usually becomes chronic.

5.36
(a)   TRUE
(b)   FALSE   –   It occurs most commonly in children. Highest incidence at 3–4 years of age.
(c)   TRUE   –   The disease is recognized when these exceed 4% (> 10^8 cells) of the cell total.
(d)   FALSE   –   There is a proliferation of myeloblasts.
(e)   FALSE   –   Various chromosome abnormalities are seen in 50% of cases.

5.37
(a)   FALSE   –   Pallor is common due to anaemia.
(b)   TRUE   –   Bleeding tendency due to thrombocytopenia.
(c)   TRUE   –   Fever secondary to widespread infection secondary to neutropenia.
(d)   TRUE   –   Moderate splenomegaly. Hepatomegaly especially in ALL.
(e)   FALSE   –   These are the red spots seen on the trunk which increase in numbers with normal ageing.

5.38
(a)   FALSE   –   At least three cytotoxics are used in combination to increase effect and reduce possibility of drug resistance.
(b)   FALSE
(c)   FALSE   –   Platelet concentrates are used for bleeding in the presence of thrombocytopenia (usually < 20×10^9/l). Septicaemia is treated with barrier nursing, intravenous antibiotics and leucocyte concentrates.
(d)   TRUE   –   In CNS and testicular involvement in ALL.
(e)   TRUE

5.39
(a)   FALSE   –   Prognosis is best in children (median survival = 60 months compared with 18 months in the adult).
(b)   TRUE
(c)   TRUE   –   Associated with poorer prognosis.
(d)   FALSE   –   ALL is classified on the presence of immunological markers into common non-T, non-B ALL which show a antigen and null-ALL (non-T, non-B) which do not.
(e)   FALSE

5.40
(a)   FALSE   –   Median survival is 12–18 months.
(b)   TRUE
(c)   TRUE
(d)   FALSE   –   Thrombocytopenia occurs and can be severe.
(e)   FALSE   –   Rarely in older patients it may run a subacute course.

5.41 The following are features of tumour lysis syndrome:
(a) Hyperuricaemia.
(b) Hypercalcaemia.
(c) Hyperphosphataemia.
(d) Hypokalaemia.
(e) A low urea.

5.42 The following are possible complications of blood transfusion:
(a) Iron deficiency anaemia.
(b) Cytomegalovirus infection.
(c) Hypokalaemia.
(d) Haemolysis.
(e) Bleeding.

5.43 The following are associated with a hyperviscosity syndrome:
(a) Polycythaemia rubra vera.
(b) Pernicious anaemia.
(c) Hypothyroidism.
(d) Hypovolaemic shock.
(e) Sickle cell disease.

5.44 The following are indications for bone marrow transplantation:
(a) ALL in relapse.
(b) AML in remission.
(c) Severe aplastic anaemia.
(d) Thalassaemia.
(e) Normochromic normocytic anaemia.

5.45 Regarding chronic granulocytic (myeloid) leukaemia (CGL):
(a) It commonly transforms terminally into an acute leukaemia.
(b) It is more common in children.
(c) Systemic features are common.
(d) The bone marrow is hypocellular.
(e) Serum B_{12} is raised.

5.41
(a)	TRUE	– Usually > 1.2 mmol/l.
(b)	FALSE	– Usually hypocalcaemia.
(c)	TRUE	
(d)	FALSE	– Hyperkalaemia occurs.
(e)	FALSE	– Raised creatinine and blood urea.

This is due to the rapid destruction of tumour cells by cytotoxic therapy especially with undifferentiated lymphomas and ALL.

5.42
(a)	FALSE	– Iron overload occurs with recurrent transfusions (> 100 units).
(b)	TRUE	– This is a late complication.
(c)	FALSE	– Hyperkalaemia occurs more commonly.
(d)	TRUE	– With mismatched transfusions.
(e)	TRUE	– Due to clotting abnormalities with transfusion of multiple units.

5.43
(a)	TRUE
(b)	FALSE
(c)	FALSE
(d)	TRUE
(e)	TRUE

5.44
(a)	FALSE	– During remission especially if there is an identical twin.
(b)	TRUE	
(c)	TRUE	
(d)	TRUE	
(e)	FALSE	

5.45
(a)	TRUE	– In 70% of cases.
(b)	FALSE	– Peak incidence at 50–60 years of age.
(c)	TRUE	– Weight loss, anorexia, night sweats.
(d)	FALSE	– Hypercellular with granulocytic predominance. All types of myeloid cells are found in the peripheral blood.
(e)	TRUE	– Due to production of B_{12}-binding protein transcobalamin by granulocytes.

5.46 Philadelphia chromosome:
(a) May be present in chronic myelomonocytic leukaemia.
(b) May be present in chronic granulocytic leukaemia.
(c) May be present in chronic lymphocytic leukaemia.
(d) May be present in adult ALL.
(e) Is an acquired abnormality.

5.47 Chronic granulocytic leukaemia (CGL) is associated with:
(a) Splenomegaly.
(b) High neutrophil alkaline phosphatase.
(c) Megaloblastic anaemia.
(d) Leucopenia.
(e) Median survival of 6 months.

5.48 Chronic lymphocytic leukaemia (CLL):
(a) Occurs mainly in the elderly.
(b) May be asymptomatic.
(c) May be associated with an autoimmune haemolytic anaemia.
(d) Is associated with increased serum immunoglobulins.
(e) Is associated with a thrombocythaemia.

5.49 Regarding CLL:
(a) Treatment with chlorambucil is indicated for stage 0 (absolute lymphocytosis $> 15 \times 10^9/l$).
(b) Steroids are indicated for thrombocytopenia.
(c) Transformation to acute leukaemia occurs late in the disease.
(d) Serum B_{12} is raised.
(e) Prognosis is better than with CGL.

5.50 The following are clinical features of Hodgkin's disease:
(a) Pel–Ebstein fever.
(b) Koilonychia.
(c) Splenomegaly.
(d) Lymphadenopathy involving one lymph node area is stage IV disease.
(e) Pruritis.

5.46

(a)	FALSE	–	It resembles CGL but total leucocyte count is lower and absolute monocyte count is raised.
(b)	TRUE	–	Almost always present (>90% of cases).
(c)	FALSE		
(d)	TRUE	–	Occurs in 30–40% of cases in adult but uncommon in childhood ALL.
(e)	TRUE	–	It is a translocation of part of the long (q) arm of chromosome 22 to another chromosome, usually 9 in the 'c' group.

5.47

(a)	TRUE		
(b)	FALSE	–	This is low.
(c)	FALSE	–	Anaemia is normochromic normocytic.
(d)	FALSE	–	Leucocytosis, $(50–500 \times 10^9/l)$.
(e)	FALSE	–	Median survival is 3–4 years. Treatment is with busulphan and hydroxyurea.

5.48

(a)	TRUE		
(b)	TRUE	–	20% are diagnosed on routine blood testing.
(c)	TRUE	–	Occurs in 10–15% of cases. Direct Coomb's test is positive.
(d)	FALSE	–	These are reduced in advanced disease.
(e)	FALSE	–	Platelet count is reduced (thrombocytopenia).

5.49

(a)	FALSE		
(b)	TRUE	–	Also for autoimmune haemolytic anaemia.
(c)	FALSE	–	This does not occur, unlike CGL.
(d)	FALSE		
(e)	TRUE	–	Those with stage 0 survive for 10 years. Median survival is 3–5 years. Death is usually due to infection due to bone marrow failure.

5.50

(a)	TRUE	–	Occurs in 30% of cases. It may be continuous or cyclical (Pel–Ebstein).
(b)	FALSE		
(c)	TRUE	–	Occurs in 50%. The liver may be enlarged if involved in disease.
(d)	FALSE	–	This is stage I. Stage IV indicates involvement outside lymph node areas, e.g. bone marrow, liver.
(e)	TRUE	–	Occurs in 25% of cases.

5.51 Regarding Hodgkin's disease:
(a) Tuberculosis is more common than in the general population.
(b) Hypercalcaemia may occur.
(c) Lymphocyte predominant histology is associated with the worst prognosis.
(d) The Reed–Sternberg cell is characteristic.
(e) It is commoner in females.

5.52 Regarding Non-Hodgkin's lymphoma:
(a) The immunoblastic type carries a poor prognosis.
(b) It usually presents with rigors.
(c) An autoimmune haemolytic anaemia may occur.
(d) It is more common in children.
(e) The Reed–Sternberg cell may be present.

5.53 Clinically Non-Hodgkin's lymphoma differs from Hodgkin's lymphoma as follows:
(a) Constitutional symptoms are more common.
(b) There may be a monoclonal paraprotein.
(c) Tonsils are more likely to be involved.
(d) The age of onset is younger.
(e) Lymphoma cells may be found in the peripheral blood.

5.54 Regarding essential thrombocythaemia:
(a) It is a lymphoproliferative disorder.
(b) Splenic atrophy may occur.
(c) Splenomegaly is uncommon.
(d) Haemorrhage may occur.
(e) Thrombosis is common.

5.55 Myelofibrosis:
(a) May be preceded by polycythaemia rubra vera.
(b) Is commoner in the young.
(c) Is associated with 'tear-drop' poikilocytes in the peripheral blood.
(d) Results in 'smear' cells in the peripheral blood.
(e) Is usually diagnosed after bone marrow aspiration.

5.51

(a) TRUE – Due to reduced cell mediated immunity. Antibody production is maintained until the later stages of the disease.

(b) TRUE – This occurs when bone is involved. Alkaline phosphatase is then increased.

(c) FALSE – This is associated with the best prognosis. Lymphocyte depleted histology has the worst prognosis.

(d) TRUE – This is a distinctive, multinucleated polypoidal cell.

(e) FALSE – Commoner in males (2 : 1).

5.52

(a) TRUE – The histological classification (Kiel classification) relates to prognosis. Broadly divided into 'high-grade' and 'low-grade' lymphomas with a bad and good prognosis, respectively.

(b) FALSE – Usually presents as a painless lymphadenopathy.

(c) TRUE

(d) FALSE – Median age at presentation is 50 years.

(e) FALSE

5.53

(a) FALSE – They are more common in Hodgkin's disease.

(b) TRUE – They are commonly B cell tumours and produce IgG and IgM.

(c) TRUE – They are involved in 10% of cases.

(d) FALSE – Onset is at older age (50 years). Hodgkin's disease is most common between 15 and 30 years.

(e) TRUE

5.54

(a) FALSE – It is a myeloproliferative disorder closely allied to polycythaemia rubra vera.

(b) TRUE – Due to platelets blocking the splenic microcirculation.

(c) FALSE – It is usual at presentation.

(d) TRUE – Recurrent haemorrhage and thrombosis are the principal clinical features.

(e) TRUE

5.55

(a) TRUE – 30% of cases.

(b) FALSE

(c) TRUE – These are tear-shaped red cells. There may also be a leucoerythroblastic picture.

(d) FALSE – These occur in CLL.

(e) FALSE – Bone marrow is usually unobtainble due to fibrosis.

5.56 **Streptokinase:**
(a) Is produced by β-haemolytic streptococci.
(b) Is an extract of snake venom.
(c) Is an antibiotic.
(d) Is immunogenic.
(e) Converts plasminogen to plasmin.

5.57 **Regarding chronic immune thrombocytopenic purpura (ITP):**
(a) It is commoner in men.
(b) Antiplatelet antibodies are present.
(c) It is usually idiopathic.
(d) Splenectomy is the first treatment of choice.
(e) It may be associated with systemic lupus erythematosus.

5.58 **Haemophilia A:**
(a) Is an autosomal dominant condition.
(b) Is due to a deficiency of factor IX.
(c) Is associated with haemarthroses.
(d) Is more common in women.
(e) Is associated with a prolonged bleeding time.

5.59 **The following statements are true:**
(a) In acute life-threatening haemorrhage with no time for cross-matching, O-positive blood should be transfused.
(b) Whole blood should be given in chronic anaemia.
(c) Fresh frozen plasma is used for replacing coagulation factors.
(d) Human albumin is infused in the treatment of nephrotic syndrome.
(e) Blood for transfusion is stored at body temperature (37°C).

5.60 **Regarding Von Willerbrand's disease:**
(a) Levels of factor VIII are reduced.
(b) It is an autosomal dominant condition.
(c) Epistaxis is uncommon.
(d) The bleeding time is prolonged.
(e) Desmopressin may be used in the treatment.

5.56

(a)	TRUE	
(b)	FALSE	
(c)	FALSE	– It is a fibrinolytic drug.
(d)	TRUE	– Allergic reactions and anaphylaxis may occur. Antibodies are produced after its administration and it should not be used again if used less than 12 months previously.
(e)	TRUE	– Plasmin digests fibrinogen, fibrin and coagulation factors V and VIII.

5.57

(a)	FALSE	– More common in women aged 15–50 years.
(b)	TRUE	– These are IgG antibodies.
(c)	TRUE	
(d)	FALSE	– 80% of patients respond to high-dose steroids. Splenectomy is recommended in those who do not recover within 3 months of steroid therapy.
(e)	TRUE	– Also may be associated with CLL, Hodgkin's disease and autoimmune haemolytic anaemia.

5.58

(a)	FALSE	– It is sex-linked. 33% have no family history and probably result from spontaneous mutation.
(b)	FALSE	– There is absent or low levels of factor VIII. Factor IX deficiency is Christmas disease or Haemophilia B. The inheritance and clinical features are identical to haemophilia A.
(c)	TRUE	
(d)	FALSE	– Women are carriers.
(e)	FALSE	– This is prolonged if there is abnormal platelet function. In Haemophilia A platelet function is normal.

5.59

(a)	FALSE	– O-negative is the universal donor.
(b)	FALSE	– Packed cells are used to avoid volume overload.
(c)	TRUE	– These become depleted in massive transfusions and FFP should also be given in these circumstances.
(d)	TRUE	
(e)	FALSE	– It is stored at 4–6°C and kept for 21–28 days.

5.60

(a)	TRUE	– There is reduced synthesis of this.
(b)	TRUE	– Penetrance is variable.
(c)	FALSE	
(d)	TRUE	– Platelet function is defective and there is abnormal platelet adhesion.
(e)	TRUE	– Desmopressin increases levels of factor VIII and may be given intravenously.

6 Endocrinology and metabolic diseases

6.1 In a pituitary tumour:
(a) The commonest visual field defect is a homonymous hemianopia.
(b) Skull radiology may show a 'double floor' of the pituitary fossa.
(c) The commonest hormone produced by a secreting tumour is prolactin.
(d) Surgery is virtually always required to remove the lesion.
(e) Headaches may be the only presenting symptom.

6.2 Recognized causes of hypopituitarism include:
(a) Chromophobe adenoma.
(b) Postpartum haemorrhage.
(c) Sarcoidosis.
(d) Head injury.
(e) Radiotherapy.

6.3 In acromegaly:
(a) Excess growth hormone is secreted by the posterior pituitary.
(b) There is overgrowth of soft tissues in the skin and tongue.
(c) Approximately 10% of patients have diabetes mellitus.
(d) Postural hypotension is commonly found.
(e) Life expectancy is unaffected.

6.4 Expected findings in cranial diabetes insipidus include:
(a) Polyuria.
(b) A sex-linked recessive mode of inheritance.
(c) Urine with low specific gravity.
(d) Hypotonic urine following the administration of desmopressin (vasopressin).
(e) An increase in weight during a water deprivation test.

6.5 Characteristic features of Addison's disease include:
(a) Hyperpigmentation.
(b) Hypertension.
(c) Loss of body hair in males.
(d) Hypoglycaemia.
(e) Family history of autoimmune disease.

6.1

(a) FALSE – Bitemporal hemianopia is the commonest defect due to pressure on the optic chiasm.

(b) TRUE – Due to adenoma initially enlarging on one side of the pituitary fossa. It can also be an anatomical variation in normals.

(c) TRUE – This can cause impotence in males and infertility in females.

(d) FALSE – Medical treatment can be used, e.g. bromocriptine in prolactinomas. In some circumstances no treatment is needed.

(e) TRUE

6.2

(a) TRUE – These non-functional adenoma are the commonest cause. They may give symptoms due to an increase in intracranial pressure.

(b) TRUE – Sheehan's syndrome; this is less common nowadays due to better obstetric care.

(c) TRUE – Tuberculosis can also cause hypopituitarism.

(d) TRUE – Rare.

(e) TRUE – After surgery or radiotherapy to the pituitary gland, some degree of hypopituitarism may result.

6.3

(a) FALSE – Growth hormone excess results from the anterior pituitary.

(b) TRUE – Combined with boney overgrowth, this leads to characteristic facies with an increase in skull size, a large lower jaw, coarse skin and a large tongue.

(c) TRUE – Glucose intolerance is found in 25–30%.

(d) FALSE – Hypertension may be found.

(e) FALSE – This is reduced due to associated cardiorespiratory disease.

6.4

(a) TRUE – This can be as much as 15–20 litres per day.

(b) FALSE – In the familial form of cranial diabetes insipidus (DI) the inheritance is autosomal dominant or recessive. Nephrogenic DI can be sex-linked.

(c) TRUE

(d) FALSE – In cranial DI, exogenous vasopressin (desmopressin) corrects the deficiency and the urine becomes concentrated.

(e) FALSE – If this happens, it suggests psychogenic polydipsia with surreptitious water drinking.

6.5

(a) TRUE – Particularly in hand creases, buccal mucosa and friction areas. This is not found in secondary adrenal failure.

(b) FALSE – Hypotension, often postural, is common due to cortisol and/or aldosterone deficiency.

(c) FALSE – In males, body hair growth is particularly dependent on testicular androgen production. In women, body hair may be lost due to decreased adrenal androgen production.

(d) TRUE – Cortisol is an antagonist of insulin. Reactive hypoglycaemia can occur after meals.

(e) TRUE – Including Hashimoto's disease, pernicious anaemia and insulin dependent diabetes mellitus.

6.6 **In the investigation of chronic adrenal insufficiency:**
(a) The short synacthen test may help distinguish between those with primary or secondary adrenal failure.
(b) It does not matter in the synacthen test if the patient is on dexamethasone.
(c) The finding of normal serum electrolytes excludes adrenal insufficiency.
(d) ACTH levels can help distinguish between primary and secondary adrenal failure.
(e) Normal morning cortisol level excludes the diagnosis.

6.7 **The following are recognized features of Cushing's disease (pituitary dependent Cushing's syndrome):**
(a) Hypertension.
(b) Distal limb weakness.
(c) Menstrual irregularity.
(d) Osteomalacia.
(e) Depression.

6.8 **Recognized findings in Cushing's disease include:**
(a) Hypokalaemia.
(b) Diabetes mellitus.
(c) Low ACTH levels.
(d) Renal stones.
(e) Loss of body hair.

6.9 **In Conn's syndrome:**
(a) Hypertension is a recognized finding.
(b) Hyperkalaemia occurs.
(c) Serum renin levels are increased.
(d) Tetany may occur.
(e) Polyuria is common.

6.10 **Recognized causes of hirsutism are:**
(a) Ovarian tumours.
(b) Cushing's syndrome.
(c) Thyrotoxicosis.
(d) Polycystic ovary syndrome.
(e) Congenital adrenal hyperplasia.

6.6
(a)   FALSE – Normal response only excludes primary adrenocortical insufficiency. Depot synacthen test may help distinguish between primary and secondary failure.
(b)   TRUE – Dexamethasone does not cross-react in the plasma cortisol radioimmunoassay.
(c)   FALSE – These can be normal. Typical abnormal findings are a lowered serum sodium with an increase in urea and potassium.
(d)   TRUE – In primary adrenal insufficiency (Addison's disease), ACTH levels are inappropriately high compared with serum cortisol levels. In secondary adrenal insufficiency ACTH levels are undetectable.
(e)   FALSE – This may be in the normal range.

6.7
(a)   TRUE – Mainly due to salt retention induced by the cortisol excess.
(b)   FALSE – Proximal myopathy is commonly found.
(c)   TRUE – Amenorrhoea may also occur.
(d)   FALSE – Osteoporosis is found.
(e)   TRUE – Mania or a frank psychosis are also recognized complications.

6.8
(a)   TRUE – This can occur but is usually more marked with ectopic ACTH secretion.
(b)   TRUE
(c)   FALSE – In pituitary dependent Cushing's syndrome (Cushing's disease) the levels are increased. Levels of ACTH are usually very high with ectopic production. Low or undetectable ACTH levels are found with an adrenal adenoma.
(d)   TRUE – In up to 20% cases.
(e)   FALSE – Hirsutism can occur.

6.9
(a)   TRUE – Secondary to the increased aldosterone production.
(b)   FALSE – Hypokalaemia.
(c)   FALSE – Serum renin levels are low (differentiates primary from secondary aldosteronism).
(d)   TRUE – Precipitated by the metabolic alkalosis associated with hypokalaemia.
(e)   TRUE

6.10
(a)   TRUE – Can secrete androgens.
(b)   TRUE
(c)   FALSE
(d)   TRUE – The syndrome also includes obesity, amenorrhoea, polycystic ovaries or virilism.
(e)   TRUE

6.11 Recognized features of thyrotoxicosis include:
(a) Proximal myopathy.
(b) Sinus tachycardia.
(c) Carpal tunnel syndrome.
(d) Delayed relaxation of the ankle jerk.
(e) Palmar erythema.

6.12 In Graves' disease:
(a) Men and women are equally affected.
(b) Thyroid gland is typically nodular.
(c) Exophthalmos is found.
(d) Weight loss is inevitable.
(e) Pre-tibial myxoedema may occur.

6.13 In the treatment of thyrotoxicosis:
(a) Carbamazepine is often used.
(b) Total thyroidectomy is the usual operative intervention.
(c) Hypothyroidism may result.
(d) Atrial fibrillation usually responds well to small doses of digoxin.
(e) Orbital decompression may be needed.

6.14 Hypothyroidism may give rise to:
(a) Periorbital puffiness.
(b) Carpal tunnel syndrome.
(c) Cold intolerance.
(d) Increased sweating.
(e) Polycythaemia.

6.15 Recognized causes of a goitre include:
(a) Lithium.
(b) Cough linctus.
(c) Pregnancy.
(d) Pendred's syndrome.
(e) Hashimoto's disease.

6.11

(a) TRUE – This usually resolves with treatment of the underlying disease.

(b) TRUE – Atrial fibrillation also found, particularly in the elderly.

(c) FALSE – Found in hypothyroidism.

(d) FALSE – Classically found in hypothyroidism due to delayed calf muscle relaxaion.

(e) TRUE

6.12

(a) FALSE – Women are more often affected (approximately 5 : 1, F : M).

(b) FALSE – Typically diffusely enlarged.

(c) TRUE – Other eye signs are periorbital puffiness, chemosis, ophthalmoplegia, diplopia and proptosis.

(d) FALSE – Weight loss is common but weight may remain stable or rarely increases if the patient overcompensates in terms of food intake.

(e) TRUE

6.13

(a) FALSE – Carbimazole is the most commonly used antithyroid drug.

(b) FALSE – Subtotal thyroidectomy is performed usually.

(c) TRUE – The risk of hypothyroidism is greatest in the first year after radioiodine.

(d) FALSE – It may be difficult to treat, requiring large doses of digoxin.

(e) TRUE

6.14

(a) TRUE – The typical facies includes pallor and coarse, cold skin.

(b) TRUE

(c) TRUE – Other symptoms include tiredness, weight gain and hoarse voice.

(d) FALSE – This may be decreased, with dry, flaking skin.

(e) FALSE – Anaemia (usually normocytic, normochromic or macrocytic).

6.15

(a) TRUE

(b) TRUE – If it contains 'iodides' and is taken in large doses.

(c) TRUE – Typically a small diffuse goitre.

(d) TRUE – This is a genetically-linked disorder of thyroid hormone synthesis, associated with nerve deafness.

(e) TRUE – Characteristically a firm diffusely enlarged gland.

6.16 **In thyroid cancer:**
(a) Commonest type found is follicular.
(b) Calcitonin may be secreted.
(c) An anaplastic type is highly malignant.
(d) 'Cold' nodule may be found with radioisotope scanning.
(e) Exposure to ionizing radiation is a predisposing factor.

6.17 **Recognized features of primary hyperparathyroidism include:**
(a) Diarrhoea.
(b) Renal stones.
(c) Osteoporosis.
(d) Cataracts.
(e) Peptic ulcer.

6.18 **In diabetes mellitus, the following characteristically cause an alteration in vision:**
(a) Macular oedema.
(b) Cataracts.
(c) Retinal detachment.
(d) Glaucoma.
(e) Vitreous haemorrhage.

6.19 **In diabetic ketoacidosis:**
(a) Hypotonic saline is the fluid replacement most often indicated.
(b) Large volumes of fluid may be needed.
(c) Precipitating episode may be a urinary tract infection.
(d) Abdominal pain may be a prominent symptom.
(e) Potassium supplementation is rarely required.

6.20 **Common presenting features of diabetes mellitus in the young are:**
(a) Weight loss.
(b) Polydipsia.
(c) Vulval infections.
(d) Diabetic amyotrophy.
(e) Decrease in visual acuity due to proliferative retinopathy.

6.16

(a)	FALSE	–	Papillary type is the commonest. It tends to occur in the relatively young.
(b)	TRUE	–	By medullary carcinomas.
(c)	TRUE	–	Usually presents in the elderly and has a very poor prognosis.
(d)	TRUE	–	Due to the carcinoma having poorer function than the surrounding tissue.
(e)	TRUE	–	Usually in childhood. Exposure to radioiodine treatment for thyrotoxicosis is not a risk factor.

6.17

(a)	FALSE	–	Constipation, vomiting, thirst and polyuria are typical symptoms.
(b)	TRUE	–	Due to hypercalciuria.
(c)	FALSE	–	Typical bone changes are subperiosteal erosions (particularly in the phalanges).
(d)	FALSE	–	There is calcium deposition in the conjunctiva.
(e)	TRUE		

6.18

(a)	TRUE	–	Particularly in non-insulin dependent diabetes.
(b)	TRUE		
(c)	TRUE		
(d)	TRUE		
(e)	TRUE	–	Feature of proliferative retinopathy.

6.19

(a)	FALSE	–	Patient is usually sodium depleted and requires isotonic saline.
(b)	TRUE	–	Average deficit is approximately 6 litres.
(c)	TRUE	–	Other causes are respiratory and gut infections. Sputum, blood and urine should be cultured.
(d)	TRUE	–	Particularly in children.
(e)	FALSE	–	Total body potassium is always low, despite the initial plasma potassium sometimes being elevated.

6.20

(a)	TRUE		
(b)	TRUE	–	Other symptoms are polyuria, nocturia and tiredness.
(c)	TRUE	–	Balanitis may occur in males.
(d)	FALSE	–	This is particularly found in middle aged patients with non-insulin dependent diabetes, in whom it may be the presenting feature.
(e)	FALSE	–	Proliferative retinopathy usually presents after 10–15 years of diabetes in insulin dependent diabetics.

6.21 Osteogenesis imperfecta:
(a) May cause perinatal death.
(b) May produce blue sclerae.
(c) Is inherited as a sex-linked recessive condition.
(d) Can cause nerve deafness.
(e) Is associated with a low serum calcium.

6.22 Recognized associations of diabetic nephropathy are:
(a) Hypertension.
(b) Anaemia.
(c) Retinopathy.
(d) Cardiovascular disease.
(e) Nephrotic syndrome.

6.23 The following can cause secondary diabetes:
(a) Haemochromatosis.
(b) Addison's disease.
(c) Acromegaly.
(d) Angiotensin converting enzyme (ACE) inhibitors.
(e) Thyrotoxicosis.

6.24 Recognized complications of diabetes mellitus include:
(a) Lipohypertrophy.
(b) Photosensitivity with oral hypoglycaemic agents.
(c) An isolated cranial nerve palsy.
(d) Necrobiosis lipoidica diabeticorum.
(e) Xanthelasma

6.25 Characteristic features of hypothermia include:
(a) An association with hypothyroidism in 50% of cases.
(b) Alkalosis.
(c) General increase in voltage size in the ECG.
(d) j waves in the ECG.
(e) Bradycardia.

6.21
(a)   TRUE   –   In the severe form, particularly if multiple rib fractures.
(b)   TRUE   –   Other clinical features are hypermobile joints, multiple fractures and heart valve disease.
(c)   FALSE   –   Autosomal dominant or recessive.
(d)   TRUE
(e)   FALSE

6.22
(a)   TRUE   –   This is common.
(b)   TRUE
(c)   TRUE   –   If there is no evidence of diabetic eye disease, then renal disease secondary to diabetes is very unusual.
(d)   TRUE   –   Often asymptomatic.
(e)   TRUE

6.23
(a)   TRUE   –   'Bronzed' diabetes.
(b)   FALSE   –   Increased insulin sensitivity can occur.
(c)   TRUE   –   Approximately 10% of patients have diabetes.
(d)   FALSE   –   Thiazide diuretics can cause glucose intolerance.
(e)   TRUE

6.24
(a)   TRUE
(b)   TRUE   –   This can occur with chlorpropamide.
(c)   TRUE
(d)   TRUE   –   This can precede the onset of diabetes. It is usually found over the shins.
(e)   TRUE   –   Due to associated hyperlipidaemia.

6.25
(a)   FALSE   –   In only 5% of cases.
(b)   FALSE   –   Acidosis, and tissue hypoxia.
(c)   FALSE   –   There may be a generalized voltage decrease.
(d)   TRUE
(e)   TRUE

6.26 Peripheral diabetic neuropathy:
(a) Can result in pain, worse at night.
(b) Is found in < 5% of diabetic patients after 20–25 years of diabetes.
(c) Can result in foot ulceration.
(d) May result in an increase in warmth in the feet.
(e) Nearly always resolves with improved diabetic control.

6.27 Hyperosmolar non-ketotic coma:
(a) May be the presenting event in an undiagnosed diabetic.
(b) Is more common in the younger than the older diabetic patient.
(c) Is usually treated with normal (0.9%) saline for fluid replacement.
(d) Is characterized by a low plasma bicarbonate concentration.
(e) Has a mortality of 40–50%.

6.28 In the treatment of diabetes mellitus with oral hypoglycaemic agents:
(a) Sulphonylureas and biguanides must not be used together.
(b) Gastrointestinal disturbances are common with metformin.
(c) There is no risk of lactic acidosis with metformin.
(d) Biguanides are more appropriate than sulphonylureas for the obese patient.
(e) There is less risk of hypoglycaemic episodes with sulphonylureas than biguanides.

6.29 Causes of hypoglycaemia include:
(a) Insulinoma.
(b) Hypoadrenalism.
(c) Paracetamol overdosage.
(d) Alcohol.
(e) Hepatoma.

6.30 In a diabetic patient who is comatose, a hypoglycaemic coma is more likely than a ketotic coma if:
(a) Onset has been over days.
(b) Patient is young.
(c) Pulse is full.
(d) Breathing is deep, sighing and long.
(e) Patient is on insulin.

6.26

(a)	TRUE	–	This is typical of neuropathic pain. Other symptoms include burning or shooting pain.
(b)	FALSE	–	It is common, with up to 50% of diabetics having neurophysiological evidence of neuropathy after 20–25 years of diabetes.
(c)	TRUE		
(d)	TRUE	–	Autonomic neuropathy can result in an increased blood flow so the foot feels warm, often with distended veins on the surface.
(e)	FALSE	–	It can persist despite good diabetic control.

6.27

(a)	TRUE		
(b)	FALSE	–	Tends to occur in the elderly diabetic.
(c)	FALSE	–	0.45% saline is usually given if the sodium level is above an arbitary value (e.g. 145 mmol/l), although the exact level at which this is given is under debate.
(d)	FALSE	–	Serum bicarbonate is usually normal and ketones are usually absent in the urine.
(e)	TRUE		

6.28

(a)	FALSE	–	They can be used in combination if control is inadequate with single therapy.
(b)	TRUE		
(c)	FALSE	–	This can occur but is far more common in the presence of renal failure.
(d)	TRUE	–	Metformin is nowadays the only biguanide used. Sulphonylureas tend to encourage weight gain.
(e)	FALSE	–	Sulphonylureas can lead to hypoglycaemia, usually within 4–6 hours of taking the drug. Metformin does not have this risk.

6.29

(a)	TRUE		
(b)	TRUE	–	Hypopituitarism and hypothyroidism as well.
(c)	TRUE		
(d)	TRUE		
(e)	TRUE		

6.30

(a)	FALSE	–	Symptoms come on rapidly with hypoglycaemia.
(b)	FALSE	–	Both types of coma occur in the young.
(c)	FALSE	–	This can occur in both hyper- and hypoglycaemic comas.
(d)	FALSE	–	Air hunger is usually found in diabetic ketoacidosis. In hypoglycaemia, breathing is usually normal or shallow.
(e)	FALSE	–	Both types of coma occur.

6.31 **The following are characteristic features of carcinoid syndrome:**
(a) Flushing.
(b) Hypertension.
(c) Constipation.
(d) Breathlessness.
(e) Mitral stenosis.

6.32 **In Paget's disease:**
(a) Urinary hydroxyproline levels can be used to monitor the effects of treatment.
(b) If there are radiological changes of the disease, treatment should always be given.
(c) Bisphosphanates may induce remission.
(d) The serum alkaline phosphatase level does not reflect the severity of the disease.
(e) Bed rest may cause hypercalcaemia.

6.33 **Recognized associations of osteoporosis are:**
(a) Acromegaly.
(b) Hypogonadism.
(c) Rheumatoid arthritis.
(d) Thyrotoxicosis.
(e) Alcoholism.

6.34 **In osteomalacia:**
(a) Skeletal pain is common.
(b) Serum calcium levels are normal, with a reduction in serum phosphate.
(c) Radiography of the femur may show Looser's zones.
(d) Bone biopsy typically shows evidence of a decrease in osteoid tissue.
(e) The patient may have difficulty getting out of a chair.

6.35 **Recognized features of Paget's disease are:**
(a) Bone pain.
(b) Subperiosteal cysts.
(c) An increased incidence in females.
(d) Deafness.
(e) An increased risk of bone malignancy.

6.31

(a)	TRUE	– Symptoms of carcinoid syndrome occur when a carcinoid tumour has metastasized.
(b)	FALSE	
(c)	FALSE	– Nausea, vomiting or diarrhoea may be present.
(d)	TRUE	– Due to bronchospasm.
(e)	FALSE	– Pulmonary or tricuspid stenosis may be found.

6.32

(a)	TRUE	– As can serum alkaline phosphatase levels.
(b)	FALSE	– Treatment is not always needed and depends on site, symptoms, etc.
(c)	TRUE	– Other drugs used include calcitonin.
(d)	FALSE	
(e)	TRUE	

6.33

(a)	FALSE	– Endocrine causes are Cushing's syndrome and glucocorticoid therapy.
(b)	TRUE	– Osteoporosis is also associated with post menopausal state.
(c)	TRUE	– Producing localized osteoporosis.
(d)	TRUE	– Also thyroxine treatment.
(e)	TRUE	

6.34

(a)	TRUE	– Bone may be tender to touch.
(b)	FALSE	– Serum calcium and phosphate are both decreased with an increase in alkaline phosphatase.
(c)	TRUE	– These are found at points of stress, e.g. neck of humerus, ribs, pubic rami.
(d)	FALSE	– There is excess osteoid tissue.
(e)	TRUE	– Due to a proximal myopathy.

6.35

(a)	TRUE	
(b)	FALSE	– Characteristic X-ray changes are thickening of the cortex with thick trabeculae.
(c)	FALSE	– Males are more commonly affected.
(d)	TRUE	
(e)	TRUE	– Usually due to bone sarcoma.

6.36   Hypercalcaemia is a recognized association of:
(a)   Bronchial carcinoma.
(b)   Sarcoidosis.
(c)   Thyrotoxicosis.
(d)   Myeloma.
(e)   Hypoparathyroidism.

6.37   Hypocalcaemia is an association of:
(a)   Milk-alkali syndrome.
(b)   Acute pancreatitis.
(c)   Malabsorption.
(d)   Pseudohypoparathyroidism.
(e)   Paget's disease.

6.38   Expected findings in phaeochromocytoma include:
(a)   Sweating.
(b)   Hypertension.
(c)   Glycosuria.
(d)   Hyperpigmentation of the buccal mucosa.
(e)   Histological evidence of malignancy in 90% of cases.

6.39   Causes of hypertension include:
(a)   Acromegaly.
(b)   Addison's disease.
(c)   Diabetes insipidus.
(d)   Primary hyperaldosteronism (Conn's syndrome).
(e)   Hypoparathyroidism.

6.40   The following are characteristic features of multiple endocrine adenomatosis (MEA) syndrome Type 1 (Werner's):
(a)   Autosomal recessive mode of inheritance.
(b)   Thyroid adenoma.
(c)   Phaeochromocytoma.
(d)   Pituitary adenoma.
(e)   Zollinger–Ellison syndrome.

6.36
(a)   TRUE   – Due to metastatic bone disease or ectopic parathormone secretion.
(b)   TRUE
(c)   TRUE
(d)   TRUE
(e)   FALSE – This causes hypocalcaemia.

6.37
(a)   FALSE – Causes hypercalcaemia.
(b)   TRUE
(c)   TRUE   – Due to vitamin D and calcium malabsorption.
(d)   TRUE   – There is parathormone resistance and this usually presents in childhood.
(e)   FALSE – This can cause hypercalcaemia when the patient is immobilized.

6.38
(a)   TRUE   – Associated symptoms are headache, nausea, anxiety and palpitations.
(b)   TRUE   – This may be episodic.
(c)   TRUE   – Particularly if adrenaline is secreted.
(d)   FALSE
(e)   FALSE – Malignancy is found in approximately 10% of cases.

6.39
(a)   TRUE   – About 15% of acromegalics have hypertension.
(b)   FALSE – Cushing's syndrome can cause hypertension.
(c)   FALSE
(d)   TRUE   – Secondary to sodium retention.
(e)   FALSE

6.40
(a)   FALSE – Autosomal dominant.
(b)   TRUE   – Very rarely.
(c)   FALSE – This is associated with MEA Type II.
(d)   TRUE
(e)   TRUE   – Due to a pancreatic islet cell tumour.

6.41 **The following are normally secreted by the anterior pituitary:**
(a) Dopamine.
(b) Gonadotrophin releasing hormone.
(c) Oxytocin.
(d) Thyroid stimulating hormone.
(e) Adrenocorticotrophic hormone.

6.42 **In a diabetic patient being treated with insulin, the following may account for the development of hypoglycaemic episodes:**
(a) Increased exercise.
(b) Renal failure.
(c) Anorexia.
(d) Alcohol abuse.
(e) Steroid therapy.

6.43 **In a standard oral glucose tolerance test:**
(a) Patient should be on a reduced carbohydrate diet prior to the test.
(b) 25 g of glucose is given after an overnight fast.
(c) 2 h blood glucose level over 7 mmol/l is diagnostic of diabetes mellitus.
(d) Fasting blood glucose level of > 6.7 mmol/l is diagnostic of impaired glucose tolerance (IGT).
(e) Normal fasting blood glucose level excludes diabetes mellitus.

6.44 **The following can precipitate an attack of porphyria in susceptible people:**
(a) Barbiturates.
(b) Fasting.
(c) Phenytoin.
(d) Alcohol.
(e) Contraceptive pill.

6.45 **Clinical features of acute intermittent porphyria characteristically include:**
(a) Abdominal pain.
(b) Tachycardia.
(c) Peripheral neuropathy.
(d) Acute psychiatric disturbances.
(e) Skin photosensitivity.

6.41

(a)	FALSE	
(b)	FALSE	– Secreted by the hypothalamus.
(c)	FALSE	– Secreted by the posterior pituitary as well as antidiuretic hormone.
(d)	TRUE	– Also produced are luteinizing hormone, follicle stimulating hormone, growth hormone and prolactin.
(e)	TRUE	

6.42

(a)	TRUE	– Patient should compensate by increasing carbohydrate intake or decreasing the insulin dose prior to the activity.
(b)	TRUE	
(c)	TRUE	
(d)	TRUE	– Symptoms of hypoglycaemia may be mistaken for alcohol intoxication.
(e)	FALSE	– This would tend to increase the blood glucose.

6.43

(a)	FALSE	– They should be on a normal carbohydrate diet, otherwise a false-negative result may occur.
(b)	FALSE	– 75 g of glucose is drunk in a standard GTT with blood samples taken fasting and 2 h after the glucose load.
(c)	FALSE	– 2 h venous whole blood glucose level should be > 10 mmol/l to diagnose diabetes mellitus.
(d)	FALSE	– IGT is diagnosed when the fasting blood glucose is < 6.7 mmol/l and the 2 h venous whole blood level between 6.7 and 10 mmol/l.
(e)	FALSE	– 2 h sample must also be normal (<6.7 mmol/l) to confirm normal glucose tolerance.

6.44

(a)	TRUE	– Particularly when given intravenously.
(b)	TRUE	
(c)	TRUE	– Other drugs that can precipitate or attack are sulphonamides and griseofulvin.
(d)	TRUE	
(e)	TRUE	

6.45

(a)	TRUE	– Also vomiting.
(b)	TRUE	– Also hypertension.
(c)	TRUE	– Predominantly motor.
(d)	TRUE	
(e)	FALSE	– Photosensitivity is found in the other forms of porphyria.

6.46 Porphyria cutanea tarda (cutaneous hepatic porphyria):
(a) Does not have cutaneous manifestations.
(b) Typically presents with acute attacks.
(c) Is associated with liver disease.
(d) Does not have excess porphyrin in the stools.
(e) Is usually an inherited condition.

6.47 Recognized causes of galactorrhoea include:
(a) Metoclopramide.
(b) Prolactinoma.
(c) Bendrofluazide.
(d) Bromocriptine.
(e) Bronchial carcinoma.

6.48 Recognized side-effects of the combined oral contraceptive pill include:
(a) Thrombosis.
(b) Acne.
(c) Mania.
(d) Headache.
(e) Amenorrhoea.

6.49 Amenorrhoea is associated with:
(a) Thyrotoxicosis.
(b) Hypopituitarism.
(c) Congenital adrenal hyperplasia.
(d) Anorexia nervosa.
(e) Polycystic ovary syndrome.

6.50 The following can cause short stature in children:
(a) Hypothyroidism.
(b) Rickets.
(c) Coeliac disease.
(d) Turner's syndrome.
(e) Congenital adrenal hyperplasia.

6.46
(a)	FALSE	– Signs are mainly cutaneous, e.g. bullae.
(b)	FALSE	– There are usually no acute attacks.
(c)	TRUE	– Usually alcoholic liver disease.
(d)	TRUE	– Also no excess porphobilinogen in the urine.
(e)	FALSE	– Usually acquired.

6.47
(a)	TRUE	– Can lead to hyperprolactinaemia.
(b)	TRUE	
(c)	FALSE	
(d)	FALSE	– This is used in the treatment of certain causes of galactorrhoea.
(e)	TRUE	– Due to ectopic prolactin production.

6.48
(a)	TRUE	
(b)	TRUE	– Due to progestogens.
(c)	FALSE	– Depression.
(d)	TRUE	– Nausea, vomiting, tiredness and breast tenderness also.
(e)	TRUE	

6.49
(a)	TRUE	– Severe hypothyroidism also.
(b)	TRUE	
(c)	TRUE	– Usually causes primary amenorrhoea.
(d)	TRUE	
(e)	TRUE	

6.50
(a)	TRUE	
(b)	TRUE	– Achondroplasia also.
(c)	TRUE	– Other causes are renal, hepatic and heart disease.
(d)	TRUE	– Down's syndrome also.
(e)	TRUE	– Hypopituitarism as well.

6.51 **Secondary hyperparathyroidism:**
(a) Due to renal failure results in a low serum phosphate level.
(b) May cause osteomalacia.
(c) May be found in chronic renal failure.
(d) Is associated with phaeochromocytoma.
(e) May be caused by hypovitaminosis D.

6.52 **Hypoparathyroidism:**
(a) Can cause stridor.
(b) Is typically permanent after a partial thyroidectomy.
(c) May be associated with thymic aplasia in infants.
(d) May cause calcification in the basal ganglia.
(e) Is usually due to tissue resistance to parathormone.

6.53 **Signs in hypocalcaemia include:**
(a) Papilloedema.
(b) Grasp reflex.
(c) Convulsions.
(d) Positive Trousseau's sign.
(e) Main d'accoucheur.

6.54 **Hyperuricaemia is associated with:**
(a) Thyrotoxicosis.
(b) Starvation.
(c) Hyperlipidaemia.
(d) Hyperparathyroidism.
(e) Alcohol.

6.55 **Characteristic findings in familial hypercholesterolaemia include:**
(a) Hepatomegaly.
(b) Tendon xanthomata.
(c) No increased risk of coronary artery disease.
(d) Corneal arcus.
(e) Xanthelasma.

6.51
(a)   FALSE   -   This is increased. Chronic renal failure is the major cause of secondary hyperparathyroidism.
(b)   FALSE   -   Prolonged vitamin D deficiency may cause secondary hyperparathyroidism. The low serum calcium stimulates an increase in parathyroid activity.
(c)   TRUE
(d)   FALSE
(e)   TRUE

6.52
(a)   TRUE   -   Due to acute hypocalcaemia; more common in children.
(b)   FALSE   -   It is usually temporary.
(c)   TRUE   -   Di George syndrome.
(d)   TRUE   -   This can also occur in other soft tissues.
(e)   FALSE   -   This occurs in pseudohypoparathyroidism.

6.53
(a)   TRUE
(b)   FALSE
(c)   TRUE   -   In acute hypocalcaemia, particularly in children.
(d)   TRUE   -   Also a positive Chvostek sign.
(e)   TRUE   -   In acute hypocalcaemia.

6.54
(a)   FALSE   -   Hypothyroidism.
(b)   TRUE
(c)   TRUE
(d)   TRUE
(e)   TRUE

6.55
(a)   FALSE
(b)   TRUE   -   For instance in the Achilles tendon or over finger extensors.
(c)   FALSE   -   There is premature coronary artery disease.
(d)   TRUE
(e)   TRUE

6.56 Secondary hyperlipidaemia is associated with:
(a) Frusemide therapy.
(b) Thyrotoxicosis.
(c) Nephrotic syndrome.
(d) Regular exercise.
(e) Diabetes mellitus.

6.57 Diabetic autonomic neuropathy characteristically causes:
(a) Impotence.
(b) Stress incontinence.
(c) Hypertension.
(d) Vomiting.
(e) Constipation.

6.58 In the treatment of diabetes mellitus:
(a) All patients should initially be started on insulin or oral hypoglycaemic agents.
(b) Insulin should not be given more than twice a day.
(c) Patient should be advised to stop the insulin injections if they are ill.
(d) Patient should use the same site for injections unless infection occurs there.
(e) Patients can get prescriptions for insulin without paying.

6.59 The following can cause gynaecomastia:
(a) Hypopituitarism.
(b) Kleinfelter's syndrome.
(c) Adrenal carcinoma.
(d) Digoxin.
(e) Frusemide.

6.60 Gout:
(a) Most commonly affects the big toe in the first attack.
(b) May be diagnosed by the finding of positively birefringent crystals in joint fluid.
(c) Can be treated acutely with a non-steroidal anti-inflammatory agent.
(d) May be precipitated by trauma.
(e) Typically produces radiological calcification of the joint capsule or cartilage.

6.56
(a) FALSE - Associated with thiazide diuretics.
(b) FALSE - Myxoedema.
(c) TRUE - Other associated diseases include biliary obstruction and pancreatitis.
(d) FALSE - This can increase HDL-cholesterol levels.
(e) TRUE

6.57
(a) TRUE
(b) FALSE - Usually urinary retention.
(c) FALSE - Postural hypotension.
(d) TRUE - Due to gastroparesis.
(e) FALSE - Diarrhoea.

6.58
(a) FALSE - Non-insulin dependent diabetics should usually be given an initial trial of diet alone.
(b) FALSE - Short-acting insulins can be given with each meal and an intermediate-acting insulin once daily.
(c) FALSE - Blood glucose concentration tends to rise and usually a larger insulin dosage is needed.
(d) FALSE - Number of sites should usually be used, e.g. thighs, lower abdominal wall, upper arms.
(e) TRUE

6.59
(a) TRUE - Due to decreased androgen production (androgens inhibit the action of oestrogen on the breast).
(b) TRUE - Hypogonadism.
(c) TRUE - May secrete oestrogens.
(d) TRUE - Probably due to digoxin binding to oestrogen receptors and stimulating growth.
(e) FALSE - Spironalactone can.

6.60
(a) TRUE
(b) FALSE - Crystals are negatively birefringent.
(c) TRUE
(d) TRUE - Other precipitants are alcohol, exercise or surgery.
(e) FALSE - This is typical of pseudogout.

7 Renal medicine

7.1 The right kidney in humans:
(a) Is retroperitoneal.
(b) Lies slightly higher than the left kidney.
(c) Weighs approximately 1.5 kg.
(d) Receives its blood supply from the renal artery.
(e) Is composed of approximately 500 000 nephrons.

7.2 A normal midstream urine specimen on microscopy contains:
(a) Occasional hyaline casts.
(b) Up to four white blood corpuscles per high power field.
(c) Granular casts.
(d) No bacteria.
(e) Up to two red blood corpuscles per high power field.

7.3 In the assessment of renal function:
(a) Plasma creatinine may be increased by muscle wasting.
(b) Urinary pH of >8.0 is normal.
(c) Plasma urea levels give a good estimate of renal function.
(d) Urine specific gravity is unaffected by diet.
(e) Glomerular filtration rate of 120 ml/min is normal in an adult.

7.4 An increase in the serum urea to creatinine ratio is found in patients:
(a) With gastrointestinal haemorrhage.
(b) Who are dehydrated.
(c) With chronic liver failure.
(d) Taking tetracyclines.
(e) On corticosteroid therapy.

7.5 Proteinuria of over 3.5 g/day is a recognized finding in:
(a) Minimal change glomerulonephritis.
(b) Diabetes mellitus.
(c) Renal vein thrombosis.
(d) Medullary sponge kidney.
(e) Cardiac failure.

7.1

(a)	TRUE		
(b)	FALSE	–	Usually slightly lower than the left.
(c)	FALSE	–	150 g approximately in the adult.
(d)	TRUE	–	Usually renal artery comes directly off the aorta.
(e)	FALSE	–	Approximately 1 million

7.2

(a) TRUE – Hyaline casts may not be significant, being found in normal urine and after exercise. They can however occur in chronic glomerulonephritis.
(b) TRUE
(c) FALSE – These are almost always evidence of renal pathology.
(d) TRUE
(e) TRUE

7.3

(a) FALSE – This decreases plasma creatinine.
(b) FALSE – Urinary pH usually varies from 4.5 to 8.0.
(c) FALSE – Plasma urea does not tend to rise until renal function is decreased by 50%.
(d) FALSE – Also affected by fluid intake.
(e) TRUE

7.4

(a) TRUE – Due to an increase in protein absorption from the gastrointestinal tract.
(b) TRUE – Due to a decrease in urea excretion.
(c) FALSE – There is a decrease in urea production.
(d) TRUE – Due to an increase in protein catabolism.
(e) TRUE

7.5

(a) TRUE – This is the commonest cause of the nephrotic syndrome in children.
(b) TRUE
(c) TRUE
(d) FALSE
(e) FALSE

7.6 Recognized causes of proteinuria include:
(a) Chronic pyelonephritis.
(b) *E. coli* urinary tract infection.
(c) Heavy exercise.
(d) The Fanconi syndrome.
(e) Subacute bacterial endocarditis.

7.7 Causes of 'dark coloured' urine include:
(a) Metronidazole therapy.
(b) Obstructive jaundice.
(c) Methaemoglobinuria.
(d) Ingestion of tomatoes.
(e) Acute intermittent porphyria.

7.8 The following can cause hyperkalaemia:
(a) A combination of potassium supplements and ACE inhibitors.
(b) Addison's disease.
(c) Acute renal failure.
(d) Metabolic alkalosis.
(e) Secondary aldosteronism.

7.9 In the emergency treatment of hyperkalaemia:
(a) Dialysis may be indicated.
(b) 5% dextrose (50 ml) and soluble insulin are given intravenously.
(c) ECG monitoring is required.
(d) Oral sodium bicarbonate is given.
(e) Calcium gluconate given intravenously is cardioprotective.

7.10 Metabolic acidosis is characteristically associated with:
(a) Vomiting.
(b) Chronic renal failure.
(c) Salicylate overdose.
(d) Ethanol ingestion.
(e) Severe diarrhoea.

7.6

(a)	TRUE	
(b)	TRUE	– As can other urinary tract infections.
(c)	TRUE	
(d)	TRUE	– Tubular loss of protein (also aminoaciduria, glycosuria, phosphaturia, natriuria).
(e)	TRUE	

7.7

(a)	TRUE	
(b)	TRUE	
(c)	TRUE	– Blood, haemoglobinuria and myoglobinuria also.
(d)	FALSE	– Beetroot and dyes in sweets.
(e)	TRUE	– If the urine is left to stand it becomes dark red due to porphobilinogen.

7.8

(a)	TRUE	– ACE inhibitors can, by themselves, cause hyperkalaemia (particulary if renal impairment).
(b)	TRUE	
(c)	TRUE	
(d)	FALSE	– Metabolic acidosis causes the shift of potassium from the intracellular to the extracellular space.
(e)	FALSE	– Causes hypokalaemia.

7.9

(a)	TRUE	
(b)	FALSE	– 50 ml of 50% dextrose is given, with soluble insulin, to encourage potassium into cells.
(c)	TRUE	– Main clinical effect of hyperkalaemia is on the heart.
(d)	FALSE	– Intravenous sodium bicarbonate may be given.
(e)	TRUE	

7.10

(a)	FALSE	– This leads to a metabolic alkalosis.
(b)	TRUE	
(c)	TRUE	– Also a respiratory alkalosis.
(d)	TRUE	
(e)	TRUE	– Due to loss of sodium bicarbonate.

7.11 Pre-renal failure is a recognized complication of:
(a) Myocardial infarction.
(b) Septicaemic shock.
(c) Burns.
(d) Retroperitoneal fibrosis.
(e) Polyarteritis nodosa.

7.12 In the investigation of a patient with acute renal failure, the following would suggest a diagnosis of pre-renal uraemia rather than acute tubular necrosis:
(a) Low plasma haematocrit.
(b) Urine: plasma osmolality ratio <1.1
(c) Urine urea >330 mmol/l.
(d) Urine: plasma urea ratio >10.0
(e) Urine sodium >40 mmol/l.

7.13 'Renal' causes of acute renal failure include:
(a) Haemolytic uraemic syndrome.
(b) Prostatic hypertrophy.
(c) Malignant hypertension.
(d) Malaria.
(e) Contrast media.

7.14 Characteristic features of acute tubular necrosis include:
(a) History of severe diarrhoea and vomiting.
(b) Polyuric phase shortly after onset.
(c) Peripheral neuropathy.
(d) Casts in the urine.
(e) Small kidneys in most cases on abdominal X-ray.

7.15 In the management of the oliguric phase of acute tubular necrosis:
(a) Fluid replacement is calculated from measured losses and approximately 500 ml for insensible loss.
(b) Central venous pressure catheter helps in monitoring fluid replacement.
(c) High carbohydrate diet may be given.
(d) Fluid replacement given should normally be in the form of 0.9% saline.
(e) Haemodialysis may be needed.

7.11

(a)	TRUE	–	Secondary to hypotension.
(b)	TRUE		
(c)	TRUE		
(d)	FALSE	–	This causes post-renal obstruction.
(e)	FALSE	–	This causes renal uraemia.

7.12

(a)	FALSE	–	If this was raised it would suggest hypovalaemia, as would reduced skin turgor, dry tongue and empty neck veins.
(b)	FALSE	–	This would suggest acute tubular necrosis (ATN).
(c)	TRUE		
(d)	TRUE		
(e)	FALSE	–	Suggests ATN.

7.13

(a)	TRUE		
(b)	FALSE	–	This can cause post-renal renal failure.
(c)	TRUE		
(d)	TRUE		
(e)	TRUE		

7.14

(a)	TRUE	–	Leading to fluid loss, hypovalaemia, hypotension and consequently ATN.
(b)	FALSE	–	Oliguric phase early on, can last up to 6 weeks.
(c)	FALSE	–	This may be found in chronic renal failure.
(d)	TRUE		
(e)	FALSE	–	This is found in chronic renal disease.

7.15

(a)	TRUE		
(b)	TRUE		
(c)	TRUE	–	To try and prevent protein catabolism.
(d)	FALSE		
(e)	TRUE		

7.16 **Causes of sterile pyuria include:**
(a) Myeloma.
(b) Renal tuberculosis.
(c) Herpetic urethritis.
(d) Chronic prostatitis.
(e) Amyloidosis.

7.17 **The following are associated with both renal failure and haemoptysis:**
(a) Medullary sponge kidney.
(b) Wegener's granulomatosis.
(c) Weil's disease.
(d) Tuberculosis.
(e) Polyarteritis nodosa.

7.18 **An enlarged kidney is associated with:**
(a) Chronic glomerulonephritis.
(b) Obstructive uropathy.
(c) Medullary cystic disease.
(d) Adult polycystic disease.
(e) Wilms tumour.

7.19 **Recognized features of adult polycystic disease include:**
(a) Ovarian cysts.
(b) Autosomal recessive inheritance.
(c) Chronic liver failure.
(d) Subarachnoid haemorrhage.
(e) Hypertension.

7.20 **Goodpasture's syndrome:**
(a) Causes haemoptysis.
(b) Can cause rapidly progressive glomerulonephritis.
(c) Is diagnosed by finding antiglomerular basement membrane antibody.
(d) Almost invariably presents in females in the third or fourth decade.
(e) Is invariably fatal.

7.16
(a) FALSE
(b) TRUE
(c) TRUE
(d) TRUE
(e) FALSE

7.17
(a) FALSE
(b) TRUE
(c) FALSE – This can cause renal failure and jaundice.
(d) TRUE – Legionnaires' disease also.
(e) TRUE – Also systemic lupus erythematosus.

7.18
(a) FALSE – This produces a small kidney.
(b) TRUE – Produces hydronephrosis.
(c) FALSE – Kidneys are atrophic. Often a family history. Symptoms usually in childhood.
(d) TRUE
(e) TRUE

7.19
(a) TRUE – Cysts also in pancreas, spleen and lungs.
(b) FALSE – Autosomal dominant.
(c) FALSE – This contrasts with infantile polycystic disease.
(d) TRUE – Due to aneurysms of the circle of Willis.
(e) TRUE – Symptoms in polycystic disease include abdominal pain and distension.

7.20
(a) TRUE – This may be the presenting feature.
(b) TRUE
(c) TRUE
(d) FALSE – Most common in young adult males.
(e) FALSE – Plasmapheresis, immunosuppressive therapy and dialysis have improved the prognosis.

7.21 **The following can cause polyuria:**
(a) Diabetes mellitus.
(b) Nephrogenic diabetes insipidus.
(c) Chronic renal failure.
(d) Hypocalcaemia.
(e) Hyperkalaemia.

7.22 **Haematuria is typically found in:**
(a) Pregnancy.
(b) Henoch–Schönlein disease.
(c) Diabetes mellitus.
(d) Subacute bacterial endocarditis.
(e) Polyarteritis nodosa.

7.23 **The following may predispose to calcium stone formation in the kidney:**
(a) Renal tubular acidosis (type 1).
(b) Gout.
(c) Sarcoidosis.
(d) Hypoparathyroidism.
(e) Prolonged immobilization.

7.24 **Renal carcinoma (adenocarcinoma of the kidney):**
(a) Is bilateral in approximately 50% of cases.
(b) Almost never metastasizes.
(c) May present as a pyrexia of unknown origin.
(d) Is more common in females.
(e) Can cause polycythaemia.

7.25 **Predisposing factors to the development of urinary tract infections in children include:**
(a) Vesicoureteric reflux.
(b) Urethral valves.
(c) Diarrhoea.
(d) Spina bifida.
(e) Bladder diverticula.

7.21
(a)	TRUE	–	Due to osmotic diuresis.
(b)	TRUE	–	There is a decreased tubular response to vasopressin.
(c)	TRUE	–	Also the diuretic phase of acute renal failure.
(d)	FALSE	–	Hypercalcaemia can.
(e)	FALSE	–	Hypokalaemia can.

7.22
(a)	FALSE		
(b)	TRUE	–	Common causes of haematuria are renal stones and tumours of the renal tract.
(c)	FALSE	–	Unless there is urinary tract infection.
(d)	TRUE		
(e)	TRUE	–	Also SLE.

7.23
(a)	TRUE	–	Due to a combination of alkaline urine, hypercalciuria, reduced citrate excretion and recurrent infections.
(b)	FALSE	–	Urate stones.
(c)	TRUE	–	Due to hypercalcaemia.
(d)	FALSE	–	Primary hyperparathyroidism.
(e)	TRUE		

7.24
(a)	FALSE	–	In approximately 5% of cases it is bilateral.
(b)	FALSE	–	Can metastasize to lung, brain, etc.
(c)	TRUE	–	Haematuria is probably the most frequent presenting feature.
(d)	FALSE		
(e)	TRUE	–	Due to an increase in erythropoietin production.

7.25
(a)	TRUE	–	Stasis is the commonest predisposing factor to UTI.
(b)	TRUE		
(c)	FALSE	–	Constipation can; it interferes with bladder emptying.
(d)	TRUE		
(e)	TRUE		

7.26 **Urinary tract infection in adults:**
(a) Is most commonly due to *Streptococcus faecalis*.
(b) Accounts for approximately 1% of general practice consultations.
(c) Is best diagnosed by obtaining a catheter specimen of urine.
(d) Is confirmed by the presence of an organism count of 10 000 colonies/ml.
(e) Is more common in elderly males than females.

7.27 **Regarding urinary tract infections:**
(a) Acute pyelonephritis in the adult typically causes renal scarring and hypertension.
(b) No further investigation is needed, apart from a urine specimen, unless the patient has had more than four infections in a year.
(c) They may present as confusion in the elderly.
(d) Bacteriuria in pregnancy is a normal finding and does not usually lead to symptomatic infection.
(e) They are usually treated with a cephalosporin until urine culture results are available.

7.28 **Type 1 renal tubular acidosis (RTA):**
(a) Is a disease affecting the proximal tubule.
(b) Typically causes hypercalcaemia.
(c) Is associated with an acidic urine.
(d) Can cause hypokalaemia.
(e) Is an autosomal recessive condition.

7.29 **Post-streptococcal glomerulonephritis:**
(a) Typically occurs at the same time as the throat or skin infection in children.
(b) Causes a fall in the C3 component of complement.
(c) Typically has an insidious onset in children.
(d) Is not usually associated with hypertension.
(e) Has a good prognosis for recovery.

7.30 **Characteristic findings in the nephrotic syndrome include:**
(a) Hypercalcaemia.
(b) An increased incidence in male children compared with females.
(c) Hypoalbuminaemia.
(d) Hypocholesterolaemia.
(e) Proteinuria >3.5 g/day.

7.26
(a) FALSE – *E. coli* is commonest organism.
(b) TRUE
(c) FALSE – Only use if already an indwelling catheter or un-
              cooperative patient.
(d) FALSE – Organism counts of 10 000/ml or less may indicate
              urethral contamination only but counts this low do not
              exclude a UTI.
(e) FALSE – More common in females than males throughout life
              (except in neonates).

7.27
(a) FALSE
(b) FALSE – If there are more than two episodes in a female or a
              single episode in a male further investigation is needed,
              e.g. renal ultrasound, abdominal X-ray for stones.
(c) TRUE
(d) FALSE – Significant risk of acute pyelonephritis.
(e) FALSE – First line treatment is usually augmentin or
              trimethoprim.

7.28
(a) FALSE – Disease of the distal tubule. Type II RTA affects the
              proximal tubule.
(b) FALSE – Osteomalacia renal stones and nephrocalcinosis.
(c) FALSE – Alkaline urine: distal tubule unable to maintain the H^+
              gradient between urine and plasma.
(d) TRUE
(e) FALSE – Either acquired or autosomal dominant condition.

7.29
(a) FALSE – Usually occurs 2–3 weeks after the original infection,
              which may have been trivial.
(b) TRUE   – During the active stage of the disease.
(c) FALSE – Often of abrupt onset in children.
(d) FALSE – This is common.
(e) TRUE   – The majority will recover.

7.30
(a) FALSE – Calcium levels tend to be low.
(b) TRUE
(c) TRUE   – Often <20 g/l.
(d) FALSE – Hypercholesterolaemia commonly present.
(e) TRUE

7.31 Recognized complications of the nephrotic syndrome include:
(a) Pleural effusions.
(b) Muscle wasting.
(c) Hypoaldosteronism.
(d) An increased thrombotic tendency.
(e) Pneumococcal peritonitis.

7.32 Hypokalaemia is a recognized complication of:
(a) Secondary hyperaldosteronism.
(b) Fanconi syndrome.
(c) Corticosteroid therapy.
(d) Pyloric stenosis.
(e) Metabolic acidosis.

7.33 Hypokalaemia typically causes:
(a) Hyper-reflexia.
(b) Peaked T waves in an ECG.
(c) U waves in an ECG.
(d) Paralytic ileus.
(e) Muscle weakness.

7.34 Ureteric obstruction is a recognized complication of:
(a) Methysergide therapy.
(b) Sickle cell disease.
(c) Tuberculosis.
(d) Pregnancy.
(e) Analgesic therapy.

7.35 Bladder carcinoma:
(a) Is usually due to an adenocarcinoma.
(b) Is more common in males than females.
(c) Has an increased incidence in those with *Schistosoma haematobium* infection.
(d) Usually presents with asymptomatic proteinuria.
(e) Is almost always treated with radiotherapy in the initial stages.

7.31

(a)	TRUE	–	Also peripheral oedema, ascites periorbital oedema.
(b)	TRUE	–	Hypoproteinaemia.
(c)	FALSE	–	Secondary hyperaldosteronism leading to sodium retention.
(d)	TRUE	–	Due to increased factor VIII, fibrinogen and platelets.
(e)	TRUE	–	Increased risk of urinary tract infections and septicaemia.

7.32

(a)	TRUE		
(b)	TRUE		
(c)	TRUE	–	Increased renal loss of potassium.
(d)	TRUE	–	Due to vomiting.
(e)	FALSE	–	Metabolic alkalosis can cause hypokalaemia.

7.33

(a)	FALSE	–	The reflexes may be depressed.
(b)	FALSE	–	T waves typically flattened. Peaked T waves occur in hyperkalaemia.
(c)	TRUE		
(d)	TRUE	–	May get abdominal distension and constipation.
(e)	TRUE	–	Also lethargy.

7.34

(a)	TRUE	–	Can cause retroperitoneal fibrosis.
(b)	TRUE	–	Leads to necrotic papillae, as can (e) and diabetes mellitus.
(c)	TRUE	–	Strictures also occur in schistosomiasis, post-radiation therapy and post-calculi.
(d)	TRUE	–	Causes extraluminal compression, as can pelvic tumours.
(e)	TRUE		

7.35

(a)	FALSE	–	Usually transitional cell carcinoma.
(b)	TRUE	–	Particularly in the 60–70 year old age group.
(c)	TRUE	–	Also increased incidence if exposed to aniline, e.g. dyeing industry.
(d)	FALSE	–	Haematuria is the commonest presentation.
(e)	FALSE	–	Surgical resection or diathermy are the commonest treatments unless the tumour is invasive.

7.36 **Analgesic nephropathy:**
(a) Is associated with an increased incidence of urinary tract infections.
(b) Recovers after stopping the analgesics in over 95% of cases.
(c) Is associated with transitional cell carcinoma.
(d) Is more common in women than men.
(e) Is almost always due to aspirin therapy.

7.37 **The following drugs are nephrotoxic:**
(a) Erythromycin.
(b) Sulphonamides.
(c) Gold.
(d) Tetracycline.
(e) Gentamicin.

7.38 **Chronic renal failure is a recognized complication of:**
(a) Systemic sclerosis.
(b) Diabetes mellitus.
(c) Hypertension.
(d) Hypocalcaemia.
(e) Chronic hypokalaemia.

7.39 **The following findings would suggest chronic rather than acute renal failure:**
(a) Normochromic, normocytic anaemia.
(b) Urine specific gravity of >1015.
(c) Osteitis fibrosa cystica.
(d) Peripheral neuropathy.
(e) Brown stained nails.

7.40 **Contributory factors to the anaemia of chronic renal failure include:**
(a) Marrow suppression.
(b) Chronic blood loss.
(c) Decreased erythropoietin secretion.
(d) B_{12} deficiency.
(e) Haemolysis.

7.36

(a)	TRUE	
(b)	FALSE	– Approximately 30% of people have a deterioration in renal function, despite stopping the drug.
(c)	TRUE	
(d)	TRUE	– Most common in women aged 40–60 years. Primary lesion is renal papillary necrosis.
(e)	FALSE	– Can be due to any non-steroidal anti-inflammatory drug.

7.37

(a)	FALSE	
(b)	TRUE	– Can cause, for example, hypersensitivity vasculitis.
(c)	TRUE	– Proteinuria and nephrotic syndrome.
(d)	TRUE	– Can lead to increased urea formation.
(e)	TRUE	– Causes proximal tubular damage. If already renal impairment, can get nephrotoxicity despite 'therapeutic' blood levels.

7.38

(a)	TRUE	– Also polyarteritis nodosa.
(b)	TRUE	– Also gout, amyloidosis.
(c)	TRUE	
(d)	FALSE	– Hypercalcaemia.
(e)	TRUE	

7.39

(a)	TRUE	
(b)	FALSE	– In chronic renal failure, the urine is of fixed specific gravity (1010).
(c)	TRUE	
(d)	TRUE	
(e)	TRUE	– Other sign would be small kidneys on X-ray.

7.40

(a)	TRUE	
(b)	TRUE	– Due to, for example, impaired platelet function, repeated blood sampling.
(c)	TRUE	
(d)	FALSE	
(e)	TRUE	

7.41 **Typical dermatological manifestations of chronic renal failure include:**
(a) Hirsutism.
(b) Bruising.
(c) Scratch marks.
(d) Hyperpigmentation.
(e) Erythema nodosum.

7.42 **In the neurological examination of a patient with chronic renal failure, the following signs may typically be found:**
(a) Proximal muscle weakness.
(b) Decreased vibration sense at the ankle.
(c) Increased ankle jerks.
(d) Short-term memory loss.
(e) Impaired foot dorsiflexion.

7.43 **In the investigation of chronic renal failure, the following are characteristic findings:**
(a) Burr cells in a blood film.
(b) Metabolic acidosis.
(c) Hyperlipidaemia.
(d) Low serum phosphate.
(e) Low serum uric acid.

7.44 **In the management of chronic renal failure:**
(a) 20 g/day protein diet should be instituted in all patients at diagnosis.
(b) Carbohydrate restriction is usually implemented.
(c) Hyperkalaemia may be treated by dietary measures.
(d) Anaemia usually responds to iron therapy.
(e) Aluminium hydroxide may be used to reduce serum phosphate levels.

7.45 **Recognized complications of haemodialysis are:**
(a) Haemorrhagic pericarditis.
(b) Anaemia.
(c) Thrombosis.
(d) Impotence.
(e) Hepatitis B infection.

7.41
(a)   FALSE
(b)   TRUE
(c)   TRUE   –   Pruritus.
(d)   TRUE   –   Or pallor. Also look for tophi, xanthomata, vasculitic lesions, necrobiosis lipoidica which are skin manifestations of diseases which can cause CRF.
(e)   FALSE

7.42
(a)   TRUE   –   May be due to osteomalacia or steroids.
(b)   TRUE   –   Other sensory signs of peripheral neuropathy also found.
(c)   FALSE   –   Decreased.
(d)   TRUE   –   May also be decreased level of consciousness and intellectual impairment.
(e)   TRUE   –   Due to a mononeuropathy (or mononeuritis multiplex).

7.43
(a)   TRUE
(b)   TRUE
(c)   TRUE   –   Particularly increased triglyceride level.
(d)   FALSE   –   Tends to increase.
(e)   FALSE   –   May be increased.

7.44
(a)   FALSE   –   Very low protein diets used to be commonly used. Nowadays 40 g diets are usually adequate.
(b)   FALSE   –   Carbohydrate intake may be normal or increased to reduce the breakdown of body protein.
(c)   TRUE
(d)   FALSE   –   Tends to be unresponsive.
(e)   TRUE

7.45
(a)   TRUE   –   Heparin used in dialysis contributes to this.
(b)   TRUE
(c)   TRUE   –   At blood cannulation sites.
(d)   TRUE
(e)   TRUE

7.46 **The following would favour the use of peritoneal dialysis (PD) rather than haemodialysis in a patient with renal failure:**
(a) History of large bowel disease.
(b) Severe peripheral vascular disease.
(c) Aged over 70 years.
(d) Chronic obstructive airways disease.
(e) Recent myocardial infarction.

7.47 **Prostatic carcinoma:**
(a) Is most commonly found in elderly males.
(b) Typically produces osteosclerotic bone secondaries.
(c) Can be easily differentiated from benign enlargement on the basis of symptoms.
(d) Can cause an increased serum acid phosphatase level.
(e) Histologically is an adenocarcinoma.

7.48 **In the management of the nephrotic syndrome:**
(a) Protein intake should be increased providing serum urea is not elevated.
(b) Sodium restriction is not usually indicated.
(c) Diuretics are given to treat symptomatic oedema.
(d) Associated hyperlipidaemia should usually be treated with lipid lowering drugs.
(e) Steroids are of most clinical benefit in membranous glomerulonephritis.

7.49 **In renal bone disease, the following features are characteristically found:**
(a) Osteoporosis.
(b) Decreased alkaline phosphatase level.
(c) Bone pain.
(d) Raised serum phosphate.
(e) Metastatic calcification.

7.50 **In chronic interstitial nephritis:**
(a) The characteristic histological appearance is of large crescents.
(b) Intravenous pyelogram may show clubbed calyces.
(c) Infection is the cause in over 95% of cases.
(d) Lead may be a causative agent.
(e) Sulphonamides may be a causative agent.

7.46

(a)	FALSE	– This is a relative disadvantage to PD. With bowel disease, e.g. diverticular disease, there is an increased risk of infection.
(b)	TRUE	– Severe atherosclerotic disease may hinder vascular access.
(c)	TRUE	
(d)	FALSE	– The fluid introduced with PD may cause 'splinting' of the diaphragm.
(e)	TRUE	

7.47

(a)	TRUE	
(b)	TRUE	– Particularly in spine, skull or pelvis.
(c)	FALSE	– Can produce similar symptoms.
(d)	TRUE	– In over 50% of cases this is elevated.
(e)	TRUE	

7.48

(a)	TRUE	
(b)	FALSE	– Salt intake should be reduced.
(c)	TRUE	
(d)	FALSE	– This usually requires no specific treatment.
(e)	FALSE	– Minimal change glomerulonephritis is most steroid responsive.

7.49

(a)	TRUE	
(b)	FALSE	– This will tend to be increased due to hyperparathyroidism and osteomalacia.
(c)	TRUE	
(d)	TRUE	– Tends to be increased.
(e)	TRUE	– May cause calcification in blood vessels or produce pseudogout.

7.50

(a)	FALSE	– This would be found typically in rapidly progressive glomerulonephritis.
(b)	TRUE	– Also small, scarred kidneys.
(c)	FALSE	– Infection plays a small role in this disease.
(d)	TRUE	
(e)	TRUE	

7.51 **The following may cause loin pain:**
(a) Renal artery stenosis.
(b) Renal calculus.
(c) Pyelonephritis.
(d) Sickle cell disease.
(e) Acute glomerulonephritis.

7.52 **Minimal change glomerulonephritis:**
(a) Is a disease mainly of adults.
(b) Appears normal histologically on light microscopy.
(c) Is characterized by IgM deposition along the basement membrane.
(d) Typically presents with a non-selective proteinuria.
(e) Causing the nephrotic syndrome, if initially responsive to steroids, it does not relapse.

7.53 **IgA nephropathy (Berger's disease):**
(a) Is associated with a characteristic rash.
(b) May be associated with respiratory tract infections.
(c) Is treated with oral steroids in most cases.
(d) Typically presents with proteinuria in adolescents.
(e) Has an almost universally poor prognosis.

7.54 **The characteristic features of the hepatorenal syndrome are:**
(a) Precipitation by paracentesis.
(b) Oliguria.
(c) Proteinuria >3 g/24 h.
(d) Urinary sodium >40 mmol/l.
(e) Urine: plasma osmolality ratio <1:1.

7.55 **Testicular tumours:**
(a) Are most commonly teratomas.
(b) Arise usually in males >60 years old.
(c) Can produce a positive pregnancy test.
(d) May produce enlargement of the supraclavicular lymph nodes.
(e) Usually produce enlargement of the inguinal lymph nodes.

7.51
(a) FALSE
(b) TRUE
(c) TRUE – Also pain from perinephric abscess.
(d) TRUE – Due to infarction.
(e) TRUE

7.52
(a) FALSE – Commonest in children.
(b) TRUE – Electron microscopy shows fusion of foot processes.
(c) FALSE – No deposits of immunoglobulins.
(d) FALSE – Selective proteinuria, e.g. transferrin : IgG ratio.
(e) FALSE – Majority of children initially respond to steroids but many (approximately 50%) will relapse.

7.53
(a) FALSE
(b) TRUE
(c) FALSE – No treatment usually needed.
(d) FALSE – Usually presents with haematuria in young males.
(e) FALSE – Prognosis is very good.

7.54
(a) TRUE – Can also be precipitated by diuretics or shunt surgery in person with liver disease.
(b) TRUE
(c) FALSE – Usually none.
(d) FALSE – Urine sodium <10 mmol/l.
(e) FALSE – Ratio >1:5.

7.55
(a) FALSE – Seminoma in approximately 60% of cases, teratoma 40%.
(b) FALSE – Usually in 20–40 year age group.
(c) TRUE – Due to hormonal secretion, particularly associated with a rare form of teratoma.
(d) TRUE – In advanced disease;. particularly left supraclavicular node enlargement.
(e) FALSE – Spreads to para-aortic nodes.

7.56   The following are indications for urinary catheterization:
(a)   Nephrotic syndrome
(b)   Urinary retention.
(c)   Renal calculus.
(d)   Urinary output measurement in critically ill patient.
(e)   Urinary tract infection.

7.57   Thrombotic thrombocytopenic purpura:
(a)   Occurs only in children.
(b)   Causes oliguria.
(c)   Can cause convulsions.
(d)   Is a benign condition.
(e)   Is associated with haemolysis.

7.58   Diabetes mellitus is characteristically associated with:
(a)   Nodular glomerulosclerosis.
(b)   Myoglobinuria.
(c)   Pyelonephritis.
(d)   Diffuse glomerulosclerosis.
(e)   Renal papillary necrosis.

7.59   Drugs toxic to the kidney include:
(a)   Methicillin.
(b)   Penicillamine.
(c)   Urokinase.
(d)   Biligrafin.
(e)   Rifampicin.

7.60   Complications of an indwelling urinary catheter include:
(a)   Haematuria.
(b)   Septicaemia.
(c)   Urethral stricture.
(d)   Chronic bacterial prostatitis.
(e)   Urinary tract obstruction.

7.56
(a)	FALSE
(b)	TRUE
(c)	FALSE
(d)	TRUE
(e)	FALSE

7.57
(a)	FALSE	– Occurs most commonly in 10–40 year age group.
(b)	TRUE	
(c)	TRUE	– Also coma and other neurological features.
(d)	FALSE	– Mortality up to 75% within few months of onset.
(e)	TRUE	– Coombs'-negative.

7.58
(a)	TRUE	– This is pathognomonic of diabetes.
(b)	FALSE	
(c)	TRUE	
(d)	TRUE	
(e)	TRUE	

7.59
(a)	TRUE	– Uncommon.
(b)	TRUE	– Should regularly test for proteinuria.
(c)	FALSE	
(d)	TRUE	– This is used as a contrast medium in radiography.
(e)	TRUE	– Can cause tubular and interstitial damage.

7.60
(a)	TRUE	– Due to bladder wall irritation.
(b)	TRUE	
(c)	TRUE	– Due to traumatic catheterization, or failure to change the catheter.
(d)	TRUE	
(e)	TRUE	– Due to obstruction of the catheter.

8 Gastroenterology

8.1 The following can cause hepatomegaly:
(a) Infectious mononucleosis.
(b) Lymphoma.
(c) Brucellosis.
(d) Tricuspid stenosis.
(e) Pernicious anaemia.

8.2 The following can cause splenomegaly:
(a) Idiopathic thrombocytopaenic purpura.
(b) Myelofibrosis.
(c) SLE.
(d) Polyarteritis nodosa.
(e) Gaucher's disease.

8.3 Clubbing is associated with:
(a) Irritable bowel syndrome.
(b) Coeliac disease.
(c) Diverticular disease.
(d) Crohn's disease.
(e) Cystic fibrosis.

8.4 Gilbert's syndrome:
(a) Can be precipitated by fasting.
(b) Is a sex-linked recessive condition.
(c) Reduces life expectancy by approximately 10 years.
(d) Results in a raised serum conjugated bilirubin.
(e) Results in an abnormal liver biopsy.

8.5 Recognized features of the Plummer–Vinson syndrome are:
(a) Dysphagia.
(b) Post-cricoid web.
(c) Clubbing.
(d) Deficiency of folic acid.
(e) Glossitis.

8.1
(a) TRUE – Causes slight hepatomegaly. Other viral infections associated with hepatomegaly are infectious and serum hepatitis.
(b) TRUE – Metastatic carcinoma (common) and primary hepatoma are other malignant causes of liver enlargement.
(c) TRUE – Other bacterial causes are tuberculosis and Weil's disease.
(d) TRUE – Tricuspid regurgitation more commonly causes hepatomegaly. Congestive cardiac failure (common) and constrictive pericarditis are other cardiovascular causes.
(e) FALSE – This can cause slight splenomegaly.

8.2
(a) TRUE – Other haematological causes are polycythaemia rubra vera, congenital spherocytosis and leukaemia.
(b) TRUE – Can cause a very large spleen.
(c) TRUE – Other causes are rheumatoid arthritis, sarcoidosis, amyloidosis.
(d) FALSE – But it can cause abdominal pain.
(e) TRUE – Uncommon but can cause a large spleen.

8.3
(a) FALSE – If clubbing is found in a patient with gastrointestinal symptoms, other causes of altered bowel habit must be sought.
(b) TRUE – The first sign of clubbing is fluctuation of the nail bed.
(c) FALSE
(d) TRUE – Cirrhosis of the liver is also associated with clubbing.
(e) TRUE

8.4
(a) TRUE – Can also be precipitated by alcohol, fatigue or infection.
(b) FALSE – Inherited in some cases as an autosomal dominant condition; is the only common congenital hyperbilirubinaemia. Usually due to glucuronyl transferase deficiency.
(c) FALSE – Benign condition with a very good prognosis. Treatment not usually needed.
(d) FALSE – There is a raised unconjugated hyperbilirubinaemia. Other liver function tests are normal.
(e) FALSE – Normal histological appearances.

8.5
(a) TRUE – Particularly for solids; can be intermittent.
(b) TRUE – This is pre-cancerous. Can be seen on barium swallow or endoscopy.
(c) FALSE – Koilonychia can be seen in the fingers.
(d) FALSE – There is an iron deficiency anaemia.
(e) TRUE

8.6 Recognized causes of dysphagia include:
(a) Pharyngeal pouch.
(b) Myasthenia gravis.
(c) SLE
(d) Achalasia of the cardia.
(e) Goitre.

8.7 Familial polyposis coli:
(a) Only involves the small intestine.
(b) Is inherited as an autosomal recessive trait.
(c) Is a benign condition.
(d) Does not usually present until the person is 50–60 years old.
(e) May cause bright red blood per rectum.

8.8 Chronic constipation is a recognized association of:
(a) Gastrectomy.
(b) Hyperthyroidism.
(c) Hypokalaemia.
(d) Iron salts.
(e) Hirschprung's disease.

8.9 Expected findings in idiopathic haemochromatosis are:
(a) Diabetes mellitus.
(b) An increased incidence in females.
(c) Raised serum ferritin.
(d) Hepatomegaly.
(e) Primary hepatoma in 90% of cases.

8.10 The following statements are true with regard to the spleen:
(a) It is notched.
(b) The examining hand cannot get above the spleen.
(c) Percussion over the spleen is resonant.
(d) The typical enlargement is diagonally downwards.
(e) It can sometimes be more easily palpated with the patient lying on their left side.

8.6

(a)	TRUE	–	Other causes are oesophageal inflammation, stricture or tumour.
(b)	TRUE	–	Bulbar and pseudobulbar palsy as well.
(c)	FALSE	–	Systemic sclerosis is a connective tissue disease that causes dysphagia.
(d)	TRUE		
(e)	TRUE	–	Due to external compression, as can malignant lymphadenopathy, aneurysm or bronchial carcinoma.

8.7

(a)	FALSE	–	This involves the colon and rectum.
(b)	FALSE	–	Autosomal dominant condition.
(c)	FALSE	–	Polyps become malignant (after approximately 15 years)
(d)	FALSE	–	Polyps can be seen by radiological or endoscopic investigation, from the mid-teens onwards in affected families.
(e)	TRUE		

8.8

(a)	FALSE	–	This can cause diarrhoea.
(b)	FALSE	–	Hypothyroidism is associated with this. Thyrotoxicosis can cause diarrhoea.
(c)	TRUE	–	Other biochemical abnormalities associated with constipation include hypercalcaemia.
(d)	TRUE	–	As well as opiates and anticholinergic drugs.
(e)	TRUE	–	Due to a congenital absence of the myenteric nerve plexus in the distal colon and upper rectum.

8.9

(a)	TRUE	–	In approximately 80% of cases.
(b)	FALSE	–	It is more common in males.
(c)	TRUE	–	Raised serum iron and increased saturation of iron-binding capacity.
(d)	TRUE	–	Iron is deposited mainly in the liver, heart and pancreas.
(e)	FALSE	–	In approximately 20% of cases.

8.10

(a)	TRUE		
(b)	TRUE	–	This contrasts with the kidney.
(c)	FALSE	–	Dull.
(d)	TRUE		
(e)	FALSE	–	Lying the patient on the right side sometimes helps to palpate the spleen.

8.11 **Characteristic radiographic features in ulcerative colitis are:**
(a) Widening of the retrorectal space.
(b) 'Hosepipe' appearance.
(c) Shortening and narrowing of the colon.
(d) 'Rose thorn' ulceration.
(e) Pseudopolyps.

8.12 **Recognized complications of ulcerative colitis include:**
(a) Erythema nodosum.
(b) Leg ulcers.
(c) Sclerosing cholangitis.
(d) Iritis.
(e) Arthropathy.

8.13 **The following are components of the Zollinger–Ellison syndrome:**
(a) Peptic ulceration.
(b) Decrease in gastric acid secretion.
(c) Decreased gastrin levels.
(d) Diarrhoea.
(e) Pancreatic adenoma.

8.14 **In irritable bowel syndrome:**
(a) Altered bowel habit may occur.
(b) Males are more commonly affected than females.
(c) Iron deficiency anaemia is present in 10–20% of cases.
(d) C-reactive protein is usually elevated.
(e) Symptoms may respond to bulking agents.

8.15 **Side-effects of sulphasalazine are:**
(a) Nausea.
(b) Rashes.
(c) Male infertility.
(d) Neutropenia.
(e) Hepatitis.

8.11

(a)	TRUE	
(b)	TRUE	– Due to loss of the normal haustral pattern.
(c)	TRUE	
(d)	FALSE	– This is characteristic of Crohn's disease. Ulcers are typically undermined in ulcerative colitis.
(e)	TRUE	

8.12

(a)	TRUE	– This may precede diarrhoea.
(b)	TRUE	
(c)	TRUE	– Other liver complications include fatty infiltration, chronic active hepatitis and liver abscess.
(d)	TRUE	– Also episcleritis.
(e)	TRUE	– This usually involves large joints.

8.13

(a)	TRUE	– There are duodenal and jejunal ulcers, often multiple.
(b)	FALSE	– There is a marked increase in the volume of gastric acid production.
(c)	FALSE	– This is increased.
(d)	TRUE	– Steatorrhoea can also occur.
(e)	TRUE	– Although sometimes the adenoma is found in the stomach wall.

8.14

(a)	TRUE	– Other features include abdominal pain eased by defaecation and bloating.
(b)	FALSE	– Females are more commonly affected.
(c)	FALSE	– If this is found other causes of the symptoms must be found, e.g. carcinoma.
(d)	FALSE	– If this is elevated further investigations are indicated to exclude more serious pathology.
(e)	TRUE	– For instance, bran.

8.15

(a)	TRUE	– Anorexia and vomiting can also be present.
(b)	TRUE	– Hypersensitivity rash, related to the sulphonamide component.
(c)	TRUE	– Oligospermia and reduced sperm motility.
(d)	TRUE	
(e)	TRUE	– Rarely.

8.16 In coeliac disease:
(a) There is an association with the histocompatability antigen HLAB8.
(b) Rice cannot be eaten.
(c) First symptoms nearly always present at <10 years of age.
(d) Histology may show subtotal villous atrophy.
(e) There is an increased risk of leukaemia.

8.17 Recognized causes of malabsorption are:
(a) Primary biliary cirrhosis.
(b) Acute pancreatitis.
(c) Crohn's disease.
(d) Systemic sclerosis.
(e) Tropical sprue.

8.18 Characteristic features of malabsorption are:
(a) Peripheral neuropathy.
(b) Erythema multiforme.
(c) Waddling gait.
(d) Peripheral oedema.
(e) Clubbing.

8.19 Carcinoma of the stomach:
(a) Affects predominantly the fundus.
(b) Has a 70% 5 year survival rate.
(c) Is associated with blood group A.
(d) Is associated with acanthosis nigricans.
(e) Is more common in pernicious anaemia.

8.20 The following are common causes of upper gastrointestinal bleeding:
(a) Duodenal ulcer.
(b) Familial polyposis coli.
(c) Mallory–Weiss tear.
(d) Ranitidine.
(e) Ulcerative colitis.

8.16
(a) TRUE
(b) FALSE – Cannot eat wheat, barley, rye or occasionally oats.
(c) FALSE – Can present in adult life. It is being increasingly diagnosed in the elderly.
(d) TRUE – Mucosa appears flat, although sometimes short, wide villi are seen.
(e) FALSE – There is an increased risk of gut lymphoma or carcinoma.

8.17
(a) TRUE – Due to bile salt deficiency.
(b) FALSE – Chronic pancreatitis, pancreatic carcinoma and cystic fibrosis can cause malabsorption.
(c) TRUE – In disease localized to the ileum, bile acids cannot be reabsorbed. With more extensive disease there is more widespread malabsorption.
(d) TRUE – Other diseases affecting the mucosa include Whipple's disease, amyloidosis and lymphosarcoma.
(e) TRUE – This occurs particularly in Europeans who have been to or live in Asia.

8.18
(a) TRUE – May be secondary to B_{12} deficiency or associated with the underlying disease causing malabsorption.
(b) FALSE – Dermatitis herpetiformis may occur in coeliac disease.
(c) TRUE – Due to osteomalacia (calcium and vitamin D deficiency). Rickets may occur in children.
(d) TRUE – Secondary to hypoproteinaemia.
(e) TRUE

8.19
(a) FALSE – Pylorus and antrum are mainly involved.
(b) FALSE – Prognosis is poor (approximately 20% 5 year survival).
(c) TRUE
(d) TRUE – This may occur in other intra-abdominal malignancies.
(e) TRUE

8.20
(a) TRUE – This is probably the commonest cause.
(b) FALSE – This involves the colon and rectum and may cause lower gastrointestinal bleeding.
(c) TRUE – This is a tear at the lower end of the oesophagus due to continued vomiting.
(d) FALSE
(e) FALSE – This involves the colon and rectum.

8.21 **The following are common causes of lower gastrointestinal bleeding:**
(a) Diverticulitis.
(b) Angiodysplasia.
(c) Carcinoma of stomach.
(d) Peutz–Jeghers syndrome.
(e) Carcinoma of rectum.

8.22 **Regarding omeprazole:**
(a) It is an H_2-receptor antagonist.
(b) It is used in the treatment of coeliac disease.
(c) It is effective in the treatment of erosive oesophagitis.
(d) It is given four times daily with food.
(e) Gynaecomastia is a side-effect.

8.23 **The following drugs are stimulant laxatives:**
(a) Senna.
(b) Ispaghula husk.
(c) Lactulose.
(d) Loperamide.
(e) Liquid paraffin.

8.24 **A chronic gastric ulcer:**
(a) Most commonly occurs on the greater curve of the stomach.
(b) Is less common in professionals.
(c) Causes abdominal pain.
(d) Is treated by a Billroth I gastrectomy in the first instance.
(e) May be malignant.

8.25 **The following are complications of a chronic duodenal ulcer:**
(a) Malignant change.
(b) Hour-glass stomach.
(c) Pyloric stenosis.
(d) Haemorrhage.
(e) Erythema nodosum.

8.21
(a)   TRUE   – Can occur but is uncommon.
(b)   TRUE   – Angiodysplasia can occur throughout the gastrointestinal tract particularly in the elderly.
(c)   TRUE
(d)   FALSE – This is a polyposis involving the stomach and small intestine.
(e)   TRUE

8.22
(a)   FALSE – It is a proton pump inhibitor.
(b)   FALSE
(c)   TRUE
(d)   FALSE – It is usually given once a day.
(e)   FALSE – This may occur with H_2-antagonists.

8.23
(a)   TRUE
(b)   FALSE – This increases faecal bulk.
(c)   FALSE – This is an osmotic laxative. It retains water in the bowel.
(d)   FALSE – This is an anticholinergic drug which causes constipation and is used in the treatment of diarrhoea.
(e)   FALSE – This is a faecal softner. It may cause malabsorption of fat soluble vitamins and lead to granuloma formulation in mesenteric lymph nodes. Aspiration can produce lipoid pneumonia. Its use should be avoided.

8.24
(a)   FALSE – Two-thirds are found in the lesser curve and posterior walls of stomach.
(b)   TRUE   – They tend to be commoner in the unskilled and those living in poor social circumstances.
(c)   TRUE
(d)   FALSE – Treated medically with H_2-antagonists in the first instance. Many operations are available each with their advantages and disadvantages.
(e)   TRUE

8.25
(a)   FALSE – This never occurs.
(b)   FALSE – This may be a complication of a gastric ulcer.
(c)   TRUE   – This may also arise from pre-pyloric ulceration or gastric cancer.
(d)   TRUE
(e)   FALSE

8.26 **The following are classical features of a perforated duodenal ulcer:**
(a) Increased bowel sounds.
(b) Free gas under the diaphragm on a supine abdominal film.
(c) Pneumomediastinum.
(d) Abdominal rebound tenderness.
(e) Backache.

8.27 **The following statements are correct:**
(a) Vitamin C is a fat soluble vitamin.
(b) Vitamin B_{12} is absorbed in the proximal ileum.
(c) C-14 glycocholic acid breath test measures small bowel bacteria overgrowth.
(d) Duodenal ulcers are commoner in women.
(e) Thyrotoxicosis may cause malabsorption.

8.28 **Congenital aganglionosis (Hirschsprung's disease):**
(a) Is due to a congenital absence of ganglion cells in the intramural plexus of the bowel wall.
(b) Is more common in girls.
(c) Affects the stomach and duodenum.
(d) May be cured by Swenson's procedure.
(e) Results in diarrhoea.

8.29 **Regarding Crohn's disease:**
(a) It is a disease confined to the terminal ileum.
(b) Kveim test may be positive.
(c) It is more common in women.
(d) Gallstones are more common than in the general population.
(e) Osteomalacia may occur.

8.30 **The following may be associated with Crohn's disease:**
(a) Anal fissure.
(b) Aortic stenosis.
(c) Uveitis.
(d) Arthritis.
(e) Acanthosis nigricans.

8.26
(a)   FALSE – Bowel sounds are absent.
(b)   FALSE – There is free gas seen on an *erect* abdominal film or chest X-ray.
(c)   FALSE
(d)   TRUE
(e)   FALSE – This is uncommon as perforations are usually anterior.

8.27
(a)   FALSE – Fat soluble vitamins are A, D, E and K.
(b)   FALSE – It is absorbed in the terminal ileum.
(c)   TRUE   – Bacteria deconjugate bile acids which in this test is labelled with C-14 isotope. Increased deconjugation from overgrowth results in increased amounts of $^{14}CO_2$ expired.
(d)   FALSE – Three times more common in men.
(e)   TRUE   – Due to increased gastrointestinal transit time.

8.28
(a)   TRUE   – This results in loss of normal peristaltic movement.
(b)   FALSE – It is 10 times more common in boys.
(c)   FALSE – It affects rectum and large bowel and rarely extends into small intestine.
(d)   TRUE   – This is a rectosigmoidectomy with preservation of the anal sphincter.
(e)   FALSE – It presents as severe constipation from birth onwards.

8.29
(a)   FALSE – Any part of the gastrointestinal tract from mouth to anus may be affected.
(b)   TRUE   – Sarcoidosis and Crohn's disease share some common histological features, e.g. granulomata.
(c)   FALSE – The sexes are equally affected.
(d)   TRUE   – Due to ileal disease and bile salt deficiency.
(e)   TRUE   – Due to malabsorption.

8.30
(a)   TRUE   – These may be the presenting feature in Crohn's disease.
(b)   FALSE
(c)   TRUE   – Episcleritis and conjunctivitis may also occur.
(d)   TRUE   – Usually involving large joints (Rheumatoid factor is absent).
(e)   FALSE – Erythema nodosum and pyoderma gangrenosum are associated skin conditions.

8.31 Characteristic radiographic features in Crohn's disease are:
(a) Pseudopolyps involving the colon.
(b) Mucosal ulceration.
(c) Stricture formation.
(d) 'Skip lesions'.
(e) Loss of the haustral pattern.

8.32 Ischaemic colitis:
(a) Characteristically involves the sigmoid colon.
(b) Is more common in the 20–30 year age group.
(c) Results in a thumb printing abnormality on barium enema.
(d) May result from a mesenteric embolus.
(e) Usually presents with haematemesis.

8.33 Regarding cimetidine:
(a) It is a histamine receptor agonist.
(b) It inhibits the secretion of gastrin.
(c) Oligospermia may occcur.
(d) Gynaecomastia may occur.
(e) Ulcer healing rates approach 100%.

8.34 The following are accepted indications for a liver biopsy:
(a) Diagnosis of secondary tumour deposits.
(b) Hydatid disease.
(c) Coagulation disorder of unknown aetiology.
(d) Diagnosis of systemic disease.
(e) Obstructive jaundice.

8.35 The following are possible complications of a liver biopsy:
(a) Pneumothorax.
(b) Biliary peritonitis.
(c) Myocardial infarction.
(d) Gastrointestinal haemorrhage.
(e) Bowel perforation.

8.31

(a)	FALSE	–	This appearance is associated with ulcerative colitis.
(b)	TRUE	–	This may be deep and barium may enter deep into the bowel wall, 'rose thorn' ulcers.
(c)	TRUE	–	This is called the 'string sign' when it involves the terminal ileum and there is usually proximal dilatation.
(d)	TRUE	–	Lesions are multiple but there is often normal bowel in between.
(e)	FALSE	–	This occurs in ulcerative colitis.

8.32

(a)	FALSE	–	Splenic flexure is characteristically involved as the arterial supply is most precarious here.
(b)	FALSE	–	More common in over 50 years of age.
(c)	TRUE	–	This is due to oedematous swelling.
(d)	TRUE	–	If severe gangrene of the bowel will result.
(e)	FALSE	–	Usually presents with acute abdominal pain and rectal bleeding and diarrhoea.

8.33

(a)	FALSE	–	It is a histamine type-2-receptor antagonist.
(b)	FALSE	–	It inhibits secretion of gastric acid by the gastric parietal cells.
(c)	TRUE	–	This is reversible.
(d)	TRUE	–	This is reversible.
(e)	FALSE	–	Healing rates are 70–80%. Relapse is reduced by long-term treatment with 400 mg of cimetidine nocte.

8.34

(a)	TRUE		
(b)	FALSE	–	This is a contraindication to liver biopsy.
(c)	FALSE	–	There is a risk of haemorrhage even if there is no clotting abnormality.
(d)	TRUE		
(e)	FALSE	–	This is a contraindication.

8.35

(a)	TRUE		
(b)	TRUE	–	This can be fatal.
(c)	FALSE		
(d)	FALSE	–	Haemorrhage may occur from the liver which may be fatal and the patient should have blood grouped and saved before the procedure.
(e)	TRUE	–	Kidney and gall bladder may also be inadvertently biopsied.

8.36 The following are clinical features of ascites:
(a) Everted umbilicus.
(b) Caput medusae.
(c) Absent bowel sounds.
(d) Shifting dullness.
(e) Grey–Turner's sign.

8.37 The following are common causes of ascites:
(a) Pulmonary fibrosis.
(b) Congestive heart failure.
(c) Nephrotic syndrome.
(d) Coeliac disease.
(e) Liver metastases.

8.38 The following are causes of acute pancreatitis:
(a) Hypocalcaemia.
(b) Gall stones.
(c) Alcohol.
(d) Corticosteroids.
(e) Mumps virus.

8.39 Regarding oesophageal carcinoma:
(a) Adenocarcinoma involving the upper third of the oesophagus is the most common.
(b) It is associated with Tylosis.
(c) It is more common in women.
(d) It is more common in China than Europe.
(e) Gives rise to a 'rat's-tail' appearance on barium swallow.

8.40 Carcinoid tumours:
(a) Are most commonly found in the appendix.
(b) Secrete gastrin.
(c) Are associated with flushing.
(d) Secrete serotonin.
(e) Are associated with aortic stenosis.

8.36
(a) TRUE   – Abdomen is distended.
(b) FALSE – This is a sign of raised portal pressure.
(c) FALSE – Bowel sounds are normal.
(d) TRUE
(e) FALSE – This is bruising in the flanks seen in acute pancreatitis.

8.37
(a) FALSE
(b) TRUE   – This results in a transudate (<30 g/l of protein).
(c) TRUE   – This results in a transudate.
(d) FALSE – Unless it is associated with severe malnutrition and hypoproteinaemia which is uncommon.
(e) TRUE   – This and alcoholic cirrhosis are the commonest causes of ascites.

8.38
(a) FALSE – Usually hypercalcaemia.
(b) TRUE   – One of the commonest causes.
(c) TRUE   – One of the commonest causes.
(d) TRUE
(e) TRUE

8.39
(a) FALSE – Most tumours involve the lower third and are squamous. Adenocarcinoma of the lower end of the oesophagus should be considered a primary gastric tumour.
(b) TRUE   – This is a rare autosomal dominant condition also associated with dyskeratosis of the soles of the feet and palms of the hands.
(c) FALSE
(d) TRUE
(e) TRUE

8.40
(a) TRUE   – They may also occur elsewhere in the gastrointestinal tract and in the lung and ovary.
(b) FALSE
(c) TRUE
(d) TRUE   – They may also secrete kallikrein and bradykinin. Clinical features occur with massive secretion after metastasizing to the liver.
(e) FALSE – Right-sided valve abnormalities occur, i.e. tricuspid and pulmonary stenosis.

8.41 Colonic carcinoma:
(a) Often present with altered bowel habit.
(b) Is of squamous type.
(c) Is more likely in those with ulcerative colitis.
(d) May present with a megaloblastic anaemia.
(e) Is more common in women.

8.42 The following are recognized features of pancreatic carcinoma:
(a) Diabetes mellitus.
(b) Migratory thrombophlebitis.
(c) Good prognosis.
(d) Obstructive jaundice.
(e) Polycythaemia.

8.43 A hepatoma:
(a) May be multiple.
(b) Is more common in those with cirrhosis.
(c) May result in polycythaemia.
(d) Is associated with raised serum alpha-fetoprotein.
(e) Is associated with idiopathic haemochromatosis.

8.44 The following are recognized clinical features of liver disease:
(a) Flapping tremor.
(b) Cyanosis.
(c) Gynaecomastia.
(d) Koilonychia.
(e) Spider naevi.

8.45 Primary haemochromatosis:
(a) Is inherited as an autosomal dominant condition.
(b) Results in increased skin pigmentation.
(c) Is associated with diabetes mellitus.
(d) Occurs in young (<40 years of age) men and women equally.
(e) May cause congestive heart failure.

8.41
(a) TRUE – There may be blood and/or mucus in the faeces. There may also be abdominal pain and weight loss.
(b) FALSE – They are adenocarcinomas.
(c) TRUE
(d) FALSE – There may be an iron deficiency anaemia due to chronic blood loss.
(e) FALSE

8.42
(a) TRUE
(b) TRUE – This usually involves the leg veins.
(c) FALSE
(d) TRUE
(e) TRUE – There may be anaemia.

8.43
(a) TRUE – Can be single.
(b) TRUE – One-fifth of all cirrhotics develop this.
(c) TRUE – Due to secretion of erythropoeitin.
(d) TRUE
(e) TRUE – They develop cirrhosis.

8.44
(a) TRUE
(b) TRUE
(c) TRUE – Due to increased levels of oestrogens which are normally broken down by the liver.
(d) FALSE – This is a sign of iron deficiency anaemia. Leuconychia may be present which is a sign of hypoalbuminaemia.
(e) TRUE – These are usually seen in the distribution of the superior vena cava: upper arms, neck, face and chest.

8.45
(a) FALSE – It is autosomal recessive.
(b) TRUE – Due to increased melanin production and iron deposition in the skin.
(c) TRUE – This occurs due to iron deposition in the pancreas.
(d) FALSE – It is not seen clinically in premenopausal women as menstruation is nature's treatment. It is seen post-menopausally.
(e) TRUE – Due to cardiomyopathy.

8.46 Wilson's disease:
(a) Is associated with increased serum caeruloplasmin levels.
(b) Is inherited as an autosomal recessive condition.
(c) Is associated with increased urinary copper levels.
(d) Results in Kayser–Fleischer rings.
(e) Results in Parkinsonism.

8.47 Primary biliary cirrhosis:
(a) Is more common in women.
(b) Is associated with a raised IgM.
(c) Results in hepatitic jaundice.
(d) Is diagnosed if anti-smooth muscle antibodies are present.
(e) Is a progressive disease that is retarded by cholestyramine.

8.48 Regarding portal hypertension:
(a) There is an increased risk of cerebral infarction.
(b) Ascites may occur.
(c) It is most commonly caused by cirrhosis.
(d) It leads to oesophageal varices.
(e) It is common in pregnancy.

8.49 The following may be associated with oesophageal varices:
(a) Tylosis.
(b) Hepatic cirrhosis.
(c) Haematemesis.
(d) Non-steroidal anti-inflammatory drugs.
(e) Colonic carcinoma.

8.50 The following are features of autoimmune chronic active hepatitis:
(a) Preponderance of females.
(b) Amenorrhoea.
(c) Raised serum IgA.
(d) Association with HLA B8.
(e) Response to steroids.

8.46

(a)	FALSE	– These are very low. Caeruloplasmin is a copper-carrying protein.
(b)	TRUE	
(c)	TRUE	– This is a diagnostic feature.
(d)	TRUE	– These are copper deposits on the back of the cornea seen with a slit lamp.
(e)	TRUE	– Due to copper deposition in extrapyramidal tissue.

8.47

(a)	TRUE	– 90% of cases.
(b)	TRUE	– 75% of cases.
(c)	FALSE	– It is cholestatic in type with a raised alkaline phosphatase.
(d)	FALSE	– Antimitochondrial antibodies are present in 95% of cases but are not diagnostic.
(e)	FALSE	– Cholestyramine is helpful for the itching. There is no treatment to retard the course of the disease which ends in liver failure.

8.48

(a)	FALSE
(b)	TRUE – This is common and is a transudate.
(c)	TRUE
(d)	TRUE
(e)	FALSE

8.49

(a)	FALSE	– This is an inherited condition associated with oesophageal carcinoma.
(b)	TRUE	– This is the commonest cause which produces portal hypertension.
(c)	TRUE	– Commonest presenting symptom.
(d)	FALSE	
(e)	FALSE	

8.50

(a)	TRUE	– 15–50 years is usual age of onset.
(b)	TRUE	
(c)	FALSE	– IgG is raised and DNA binding positive. There is also a Coomb's positive anaemia.
(d)	TRUE	– Also associated with HLA A1 and DW3.
(e)	TRUE	

8.51 **The following are features of fulminant hepatic failure:**
(a) Metabolic acidosis.
(b) Hyperglycaemia.
(c) It may be preceded by viral hepatitis.
(d) Disseminated intravascular coagulation.
(e) Hyperkalaemia.

8.52 **The following are recognized complications of gallstones:**
(a) Ileus.
(b) Oesophageal varices.
(c) Carcinoma of the gallbladder.
(d) Carcinoma of the pancreas.
(e) Cholangitis.

8.53 **The following are clinical features of acute pancreatitis:**
(a) Cullen's sign.
(b) Abdominal pain.
(c) Dupytren's contracture.
(d) Dysphagia.
(e) Shock.

8.54 **The following are typical laboratory features of acute pancreatitis:**
(a) Serum amylase of 100 IU/1.
(b) Hypercalcaemia.
(c) Hyperglycaemia.
(d) Raised alpha-fetoprotein level.
(e) Hyponatraemia.

8.55 **The following are associated with coeliac disease:**
(a) Erythema nodosum.
(b) Splenic atrophy.
(c) Folate deficiency.
(d) Constipation.
(e) Pemphigus.

8.51
(a)   TRUE   –   Due to accumulation of the products of tissue destruction.
(b)   FALSE –   Hypoglycaemia occurs due to disruption of gluconeogenetic activity in the liver.
(c)   TRUE   –   It is uncommon and is usually caused by viral hepatitis or paracetamol overdose.
(d)   TRUE
(e)   FALSE –   Hypokalaemia and hyponatraemia occur. Hyperkalaemia may occur if associated with renal failure.

8.52
(a)   TRUE   –   Breakdown of the gallbladder wall results in a fistula between gallbladder and duodenum. If the stone is large enough it may obstruct the ileum.
(b)   FALSE
(c)   TRUE   –   <1 in 100 patients with stones, however, develop this.
(d)   FALSE
(e)   TRUE   –   Results in fever, biliary colic and jaundice.

8.53
(a)   TRUE   –   This is periumbilical bruising. When it occurs in the flanks it is called Grey–Turner's sign.
(b)   TRUE   –   This is usually upper abdominal and severe.
(c)   FALSE
(d)   FALSE
(e)   TRUE   –   In severe cases.

8.54
(a)   FALSE –   This is usually >1200 IU/l.
(b)   FALSE –   Hypocalcaemia is the rule because calcium is lost through sequestration with fat necrosis. Intravenous calcium gluconate may be necessary.
(c)   TRUE   –   Insulin may be required.
(d)   FALSE –   Only if associated with a hepatoma.
(e)   FALSE

8.55
(a)   FALSE –   This is associated with inflammatory bowel disease.
(b)   TRUE   –   Howell–Jolly bodies in the blood are common.
(c)   TRUE   –   By contrast B_{12} deficiency is uncommon as the terminal ileum is usually unaffected.
(d)   FALSE –   Usually diarrhoea due to steatorrhoea.
(e)   FALSE –   Dermatitis herpetiformis is associated with coeliac disease.

8.56 **The following are associated with gastro-oesophageal reflux:**
(a) Partial gastrectomy.
(b) Pregnancy.
(c) Polyarteritis nodosa.
(d) Systemic sclerosis.
(e) Pharyngeal pouch.

8.57 **The following drugs are associated with impaired taste:**
(a) Penicillamine.
(b) Lithium carbonate.
(c) Carbimazole.
(d) Metronidazole.
(e) Ranitidine.

8.58 **The following are extra-intestinal features of inflammatory bowel disease:**
(a) Sacroiliitis.
(b) Aphthous ulcers.
(c) Erythema marginatum.
(d) Sclerosing cholangitis.
(e) Rheumatoid arthritis.

8.59 **The following antibiotics may cause acute hepatic cholestasis:**
(a) Penicillin.
(b) Erythromycin.
(c) Chloramphenicol.
(d) Rifampicin.
(e) Nitrofurantoin.

8.60 **Regarding gallstones:**
(a) They occur more commonly in fair-haired individuals.
(b) 90% are radio-opaque.
(c) Solitary cholesterol stones are the commonest type.
(d) They may cause no symptoms.
(e) The prevalence increases with age.

8.56
(a) TRUE
(b) TRUE – Due to increased intra-abdominal pressure causing a hiatus hernia.
(c) FALSE
(d) TRUE – Due to oesophageal immotility.
(e) FALSE – This produces gurgling in the throat and may cause dysphagia.

8.57
(a) TRUE
(b) TRUE
(c) TRUE
(d) TRUE
(e) FALSE

8.58
(a) TRUE – Occurs in 20% of cases.
(b) TRUE – Occurs in 5% of cases.
(c) FALSE
(d) TRUE
(e) FALSE – Transient, large joint arthropathy occurs in 10% of cases.

8.59
(a) FALSE
(b) TRUE } Usually associated with fever, rash, eosinophilia or
(c) TRUE } eosinophilic infiltration of the liver biopsy.
(d) TRUE
(e) TRUE

8.60
(a) FALSE – They occur with equal prevalence in fair and dark coloured people.
(b) FALSE – 10% are radio-opaque.
(c) FALSE – Mixed (calcium, bile pigments, cholesterol) are the commonest type.
(d) TRUE – In 50% of cases.
(e) TRUE

9 Neurology

9.1 Possible causes of sudden blindness include:
(a) Hypoparathyroidism.
(b) Temporal arteritis.
(c) Retinal detachment.
(d) Bell's palsy.
(e) Retinal artery obstruction.

9.2 In a superior oblique nerve palsy:
(a) Diplopia is maximal on upward gaze.
(b) Ptosis is common.
(c) Pupil is dilated.
(d) Direct light reflex is usually absent.
(e) Concomitant squint is found.

9.3 Characteristic features of a Horner's syndrome are:
(a) Partial ptosis.
(b) Enophthalmos.
(c) Dilated pupil.
(d) Increased sweating.
(e) Abducted eye.

9.4 Recognized causes of a Horner's syndrome include:
(a) Marfan's syndrome.
(b) Pancoast tumour.
(c) Carotid artery dissection.
(d) Cervical sympathectomy.
(e) Rosacea.

9.5 Characteristic features of Bell's palsy are:
(a) Hyperacusis.
(b) Complete recovery in 20% of cases.
(c) Loss of taste in the posterior one-third of the tongue.
(d) Paralysis of the lower half of the face only.
(e) Ptosis.

9.1

(a)	FALSE	–	Hypocalcaemia can cause cataract formation and therefore gradual visual impairment.
(b)	TRUE	–	Treatment of this is an emergency.
(c)	TRUE	–	For instance, in diabetes mellitus.
(d)	FALSE		
(e)	TRUE	–	Other causes are acute glaucoma, skull fracture or retinal vein obstruction.

9.2

(a)	FALSE	–	Diplopia is worse on downward gaze, e.g. going down the stairs.
(b)	FALSE	–	This occurs with a III nerve palsy.
(c)	FALSE	–	Pupil is unaffected.
(d)	FALSE		
(e)	FALSE	–	Paralytic squint occurs.

9.3

(a)	TRUE	–	Complete ptosis with III nerve lesion.
(b)	TRUE		
(c)	FALSE	–	Constricted pupil (also constricted in pontine haemorrhage, morphine).
(d)	FALSE	–	Decreased in the ipsilateral half of the head.
(e)	FALSE	–	There is no weakness of eye movement.

9.4

(a)	FALSE	–	Eye changes in this include lens dislocation, myopia, glaucoma and retinal detachment.
(b)	TRUE		
(c)	TRUE	–	Syringobulbia is another cause (rare).
(d)	TRUE		
(e)	FALSE	–	50% of patients will have other eye complications, e.g. conjunctivitis, keratitis, blepharitis.

9.5

(a)	TRUE	–	If the lesion is proximal to the nerve to stapedius.
(b)	FALSE	–	Complete recovery in approximately 80% of cases.
(c)	FALSE	–	May be lost in the anterior two-thirds of the tongue.
(d)	FALSE	–	Sparing of the upper part of the face occurs in an upper motor neurone lesion.
(e)	FALSE	–	Patient cannot close the eye: when they try the eye rolls upwards.

9.6 **The following typically cause dysarthria:**
(a) Motor neurone disease (MND).
(b) Multiple sclerosis.
(c) Guillan–Barré syndrome.
(d) False teeth.
(e) An infarction in Wernicke's area.

9.7 **Expected findings in a pseudobulbar palsy are:**
(a) Increased jaw jerk.
(c) Dysphagia.
(c) Diplopia.
(d) Emotional lability.
(e) Normal speech.

9.8 **Characteristic features of an upper motor neurone lesion include:**
(a) Fasciculation.
(b) Muscle wasting in the acute stages.
(c) More marked weakness in elbow flexion than elbow extension.
(d) Hyporeflexia.
(e) Clonus.

9.9 **In carpal tunnel syndrome (CTS):**
(a) Pain is felt at the wrist.
(b) There is weakness of finger adduction.
(c) Sensory loss is usually found in the little and ring fingers.
(d) Thumb adduction is weak.
(e) Trousseau's sign is usually positive.

9.10 **Recognized causes of bilateral small muscle wasting in the hand are:**
(a) Syringomyelia.
(b) Rheumatoid arthritis.
(c) Multiple sclerosis (MS).
(d) Motor neurone disease.
(e) Pancoast tumour.

9.6
(a) TRUE
(b) TRUE – Other causes of cerebellar disease also cause dysarthria.
             MS can cause pseudobulbar palsy.
(c) TRUE – Causes a bulbar (lower motor neurone) palsy.
(d) TRUE
(e) FALSE

9.7
(a) TRUE – Commonest cause of pseudobulbar palsy is motor
             neurone disease.
(b) TRUE
(c) FALSE –
(d) TRUE
(e) FALSE – Dysarthric.

9.8
(a) FALSE – Due to spontaneous contractions of bundles of fibres;
             found in lower motor neurone lesions.
(b) FALSE – Lower motor neurone sign.
(c) FALSE – Characteristically more weakness in elbow extension.
(d) FALSE – Reflexes are increased.
(e) TRUE

9.9
(a) TRUE – Can occasionally radiate to elbow.
(b) FALSE – Finger adduction/abduction is weak in an ulnar nerve
             lesion.
(c) FALSE – Loss in thumbs, index, middle and radial half of ring
             fingers (palmar surface).
(d) FALSE – Weakness of thumb abduction and opposition.
(e) FALSE – This is a sign of hypocalcaemia. In CTS, Tinel's sign
             may be positive.

9.10
(a) TRUE – Other features in the hand include a dissociated sensory
             loss.
(b) TRUE
(c) FALSE
(d) TRUE – In progressive muscular atrophy form of MND.
(e) FALSE – This can cause unilateral small muscle wasting in the
             hand.

9.11 **In trigeminal neuralgia:**
(a) Symptoms characteristically start in patients aged 30–40 years.
(b) Pain typically lasts for <1 min, then abates.
(c) Carbamazepine is the treatment of first choice.
(d) Surgical treatment is almost never indicated.
(e) 'Trigger zone' is often found in the precipitation of pain.

9.12 **Signs of papilloedema include:**
(a) Engorged retinal veins.
(b) Enlargement of the physiological cup.
(c) Disc margin blurring.
(d) Enlargement of the blind spot.
(e) Flame-shaped haemorrhages.

9.13 **Recognized side-effects of phenytoin are:**
(a) Gingival hypertrophy.
(b) Nystagmus.
(c) Microcytic anaemia.
(d) Acne.
(e) Osteomalacia.

9.14 **Recognized causes of a peripheral polyneuropathy are:**
(a) Amyloidosis.
(b) Sarcoidosis.
(c) Uraemia.
(d) Metronidazole.
(e) Systemic lupus erythematosus (SLE).

9.15 **The following can cause nerve deafness:**
(a) Meniérè's disease.
(b) Rubella.
(c) Streptokinase.
(d) Skull fracture.
(e) Acoustic neuroma.

9.11
(a)   FALSE   –   Tends to occur in the elderly. If <50 years old, think of other causes, e.g. MS
(b)   TRUE   –   Shooting pain for 15–30 s is typical.
(c)   TRUE
(d)   FALSE   –   Surgical intervention may be needed in intractable cases.
(e)   TRUE   –   This may be on the lips or side of the nose.

9.12
(a)   TRUE
(b)   FALSE   –   This is lost and may be obliterated.
(c)   TRUE   –   This is one of the earliest findings (particularly the nasal side).
(d)   TRUE
(e)   TRUE   –   Particularly if of rapid onset.

9.13
(a)   TRUE
(b)   TRUE   –   Other signs include ataxia, slurred speech and blurred vision.
(c)   FALSE   –   Megaloblastic anaemia.
(d)   TRUE   –   Also hirsutism.
(e)   TRUE   –   Rickets in children.

9.14
(a)   TRUE
(b)   TRUE   –   Other neurological manifestations include cranial nerve lesions.
(c)   TRUE
(d)   TRUE   –   Other drugs causing peripheral neuropathy are vincristine, nitrofurantoin and isoniazid.
(e)   TRUE   –   As can polyarteritis nodosa, rheumatoid arthritis.

9.15
(a)   TRUE
(b)   TRUE   –   As can mumps and congenital syphilis.
(c)   FALSE   –   Streptomycin and neomycin can.
(d)   TRUE   –   Vestibulocochlear nerve can be damaged within the petrous bone.
(e)   TRUE

9.16 **Typical findings in idiopathic Parkinson's disease (paralysis agitans) include:**
(a) Extensor plantar reflexes early in the course of the disease.
(b) Tremor, predominantly on movement.
(c) Marked sensory loss.
(d) Bradykinesia.
(e) Micrographia.

9.17 **Recognized treatments for Parkinson's disease are:**
(a) Selegiline.
(b) Amantadine.
(c) Levodopa.
(d) Tetrabenazine.
(e) Propranolol.

9.18 **Causes of papilloedema are:**
(a) Arterial hypertension.
(b) Vitamin A poisoning.
(c) Hyperparathyroidism.
(d) Central retinal vein occlusion.
(e) Hypercapnia.

9.19 **The following can cause extensor plantar responses with absent ankle jerks:**
(a) Parkinson's disease.
(b) Multiple sclerosis.
(c) Taboparesis.
(d) Friedreich's ataxia.
(e) Vitamin B_{12} deficiency.

9.20 **The following typically occur with a parietal lobe lesion:**
(a) Déjà-vu phenomenon.
(b) Anosmia.
(c) Grasp reflex.
(d) Sensory inattention.
(e) Some forms of apraxia.

9.16

(a)	FALSE	–	Paralysis agitans does not involve any essential reflex changes. Extensor plantar reflexes common in arteriosclerotic Parkinson's syndrome.
(b)	FALSE	–	Rest tremor: 'pill rolling'.
(c)	FALSE		
(d)	TRUE	–	Slowness in performing movement.
(e)	TRUE	–	Writing becomes progressively smaller.

9.17

(a)	TRUE	–	Monoamine-oxidase type B inhibitor.
(b)	TRUE	–	Has mild antiparkinsonism effects.
(c)	TRUE	–	Used with a dopa decarboxylase inhibitor.
(d)	FALSE		
(e)	FALSE	–	May help in benign essential tremor.

9.18

(a)	TRUE	–	Malignant hypertension. One of the commonest causes of papilloedema is an increased intracranial pressure.
(b)	TRUE		
(c)	FALSE	–	Hypoparathyroidism can.
(d)	TRUE		
(e)	TRUE	–	For instance in respiratory failure.

9.19

(a)	FALSE		
(b)	FALSE		
(c)	TRUE		
(d)	TRUE	–	Degeneration in dorsal and lateral columns and spinocerebellar tracts.
(e)	TRUE	–	Causes degeneration in dorsal columns, corticospinal tracts and optic atrophy.

9.20

(a)	FALSE	–	Typically temporal lobe.
(b)	FALSE	–	Frontal lobe lesion.
(c)	FALSE		
(d)	TRUE		
(e)	TRUE	–	Dressing and constructional apraxia and spatial disorientation.

9.21 **The following are components of the Brown–Sequard syndrome:**
(a) Ipsilateral dilated pupil.
(b) Ipsilateral loss of proprioception.
(c) Complete sectioning of the spinal cord.
(d) Contralateral loss of pain and temperature sensation.
(e) Upper motor neurone signs below the level of the lesion.

9.22 **Unilateral facial or head pain is typically due to:**
(a) Myasthenia gravis.
(b) Migraine.
(c) Trigeminal neuralgia.
(d) Posterior communicating artery aneurysm.
(e) Cluster headache.

9.23 **The following drugs are useful in the treatment of tonic–clonic seizures:**
(a) Nortriptyline.
(b) Phentolamine.
(c) Carbamazepine.
(d) Ergotamine.
(e) Phenytoin.

9.24 **In multiple sclerosis:**
(a) Prognosis is poor if the disease initially presents with retrobulbar neuritis.
(b) Disease classically progresses without remission after the initial event.
(c) Lhermitte's phenomena occurs.
(d) IgM is typically increased in the cerebrospinal fluid.
(e) Ataxic nystagmus is a characteristic finding.

9.25 **Characteristic features of diabetic amyotrophy are:**
(a) Increased incidence in male diabetics in their 20–30s.
(b) Marked calf muscle wasting.
(c) Unilateral signs only in all cases.
(d) Poor prognosis for recovery.
(e) Thigh pain.

9.21
(a)	FALSE	
(b)	TRUE	– These fibres travel in the posterior column.
(c)	FALSE	– There is hemisection of the cord.
(d)	TRUE	– These fibres travel in the spinothalamic tract.
(e)	TRUE	

9.22
(a)	FALSE	
(b)	TRUE	
(c)	TRUE	– As can postherpetic neuralgia.
(d)	TRUE	
(e)	TRUE	– Severe pain, often around the eye.

9.23
(a)	FALSE	– Antidepressant.
(b)	FALSE	– Alpha adrenergic receptor blocker.
(c)	TRUE	
(d)	FALSE	– Used in treatment of migraine.
(e)	TRUE	– Used in most forms of epilepsy except absence attacks.

9.24
(a)	FALSE	– Relatively benign presentation; may be years before next 'attack'.
(b)	FALSE	– Only about 10% of cases do this.
(c)	TRUE	– On neck flexion, paraesthesiae in limbs.
(d)	FALSE	– IgG increased in approximately 60% of cases. Oligoclonal bands in 90%. May also be a lymphocytosis.
(e)	TRUE	– Nystagmus is worse in the abducting than adducting eye.

9.25
(a)	FALSE	– Commonest in males in their 60s.
(b)	FALSE	– Wasting of quadriceps, either unilateral or bilateral.
(c)	FALSE	– Can be unilateral or bilateral.
(d)	FALSE	– The usual pattern is for a good recovery, often within 1 year.
(e)	TRUE	– This can be marked.

9.26 **The following can cause mononeuritis multiplex:**
(a) Polymyalgia rheumatica.
(b) Acute intermittent porpyria.
(c) Sarcoidosis.
(d) Leprosy.
(e) Diabetes insipidus.

9.27 **In dystrophia myotonica:**
(a) Edrophonium reduces the myotonia.
(b) Mode of inheritance is autosomal recessive.
(c) Patient may be infertile.
(d) There is a posterior column sensory loss.
(e) Myotonia can be increased in the cold.

9.28 **The following would be consistent with a diagnosis of brain death:**
(a) Absent gag reflex.
(b) Delayed direct light reflex.
(c) Absent corneal reflex.
(d) Eye movements towards the ear that ice cold water is poured into.
(e) No spontaneous respiration.

9.29 **Typical features of dementia include:**
(a) Depression.
(b) Insomnia.
(c) Thought insertion.
(d) Visual hallucinations.
(e) Poor short-term memory.

9.30 **Neurological findings in B_{12} deficiency include:**
(a) Optic atrophy.
(b) Dementia.
(c) Absent ankle reflexes.
(d) Impared vibration sense in the lower legs.
(e) Fasciculation.

9.26
(a)   FALSE   –   Rheumatoid arthritis can.
(b)   FALSE   –   Can cause peripheral neuropathy.
(c)   TRUE
(d)   TRUE   –   Commonest cause worldwide.
(e)   FALSE   –   Other causes are polyarteritis nodosa and diabetes mellitus.

9.27
(a)   FALSE   –   Endrophonium reduces the weakness in myasthenia gravis (for a short time).
(b)   FALSE   –   Autosomal dominant.
(c)   TRUE   –   Due to testicular or ovarian atrophy.
(d)   FALSE   –   No sensory loss.
(e)   TRUE   –   Also increases with tiredness.

9.28
(a)   TRUE
(b)   FALSE   –   No light reaction. Fixed pupils.
(c)   TRUE
(d)   FALSE   –   No eye movements at all.
(e)   TRUE

9.29
(a)   TRUE   –   Particularly in the early stages. Depression may also mimic dementia – 'pseudodementia'.
(b)   TRUE   –   May lead to nocturnal wandering.
(c)   FALSE   –   This is a first rank symptom of schizophrenia.
(d)   FALSE   –   This is typical of organic brain disease.
(e)   TRUE

9.30
(a)   TRUE   –   Rare.
(b)   TRUE   –   Rare.
(c)   TRUE   –   Due to peripheral neuropathy.
(d)   TRUE   –   Due to posterior column loss.
(e)   FALSE   –   Sign of a lower motor neurone lesion.

9.31 Myasthenia gravis:
(a) Is associated with a thymoma in 90% of cases.
(b) Causes distal more than proximal muscle weakness.
(c) Can cause bilateral ptosis.
(d) Is treated with anticholinesterases.
(e) Is associated with marked muscle wasting early in the course of the disease.

9.32 In acute post-infective polyneuropathy (Guillain–Barré syndrome):
(a) The cranial nerves are very rarely affected.
(b) Pain in the back may be a presenting feature.
(c) Sensory nervous system is always unaffected.
(d) Upper motor neurone signs are typically found in the legs.
(e) There is a mortality rate of over 50%.

9.33 Proximal myopathy is a recognized finding in:
(a) Polymyositis.
(b) Carcinoma.
(c) Myxoedema.
(d) Cushing's syndrome.
(e) Osteoporosis.

9.34 Characteristic findings in a cerebellar lesion are:
(a) Hyper-reflexia.
(b) Intention tremor.
(c) Diplopia.
(d) Dysphasia.
(e) Ataxic gait.

9.35 Recognized causes of cerebellar signs include:
(a) Vertebrobasilar insufficiency.
(b) Medulloblastoma.
(c) Friedreich's ataxia.
(d) Motor neurone disease.
(e) B_{12} deficiency.

9.31

(a)	FALSE	– In only 10–15% of cases.
(b)	FALSE	– Proximal more than distal muscles affected. Upper limbs worse than lower limbs.
(c)	TRUE	
(d)	TRUE	– For instance neostigmine or pyridostigmine.
(e)	FALSE	– This can occur in longstanding cases.

9.32

(a)	FALSE	
(b)	TRUE	
(c)	FALSE	
(d)	FALSE	– Lower motor neurone signs in the leg.
(e)	FALSE	– Mortality of 5–10%.

9.33

(a)	TRUE	– Weakness of pelvic and shoulder girdle muscles.
(b)	TRUE	
(c)	FALSE	– Thyrotoxicosis can, often slight.
(d)	TRUE	– Patient may find it difficult to stand up from sitting. Exogenous steroids can also cause a proximal myopathy.
(e)	FALSE	– Osteomalacia can.

9.34

(a)	FALSE	– Usually decreased or pendular.
(b)	TRUE	– Tremor increases as the target is approached. It is not worse with the eyes closed.
(c)	FALSE	
(d)	FALSE	– May cause dysarthria.
(e)	TRUE	– Patient walks on a wide base, tending to fall towards the side of the lesion.

9.35

(a)	TRUE	
(b)	TRUE	– This tumour occurs most commonly in children.
(c)	TRUE	
(d)	FALSE	
(e)	FALSE	– This causes posterior column and upper motor neurone lesions as well as a peripheral neuropathy.

9.36   Typical findings in acoustic neuroma include:
(a)   Presentation usually in the over 60s.
(b)   Upper motor neurone VII nerve palsy.
(c)   Nystagmus.
(d)   Loss of the corneal reflex.
(e)   Tinnitus.

9.37   The following can cause dementia:
(a)   Intracranial tumour.
(b)   Chronic renal failure.
(c)   Hypothyroidism.
(d)   Arsenic.
(e)   Normal pressure hydrocephalus.

9.38   Thiamine deficiency is associated with:
(a)   Ophthalmoplegia.
(b)   Confabulation.
(c)   Nystagmus.
(d)   Peripheral neuropathy.
(e)   Ataxia.

9.39   The following are typical clinical features of the lateral medullary syndrome:
(a)   Hiccuping.
(b)   Ipsilateral loss of pain and temperature sensation in the body.
(c)   Ipsilateral Horner's syndrome.
(d)   Nystagmus.
(e)   Ipsilateral palatal paralysis.

9.40   In a subarachnoid haemorrhage:
(a)   Consciousness is lost in nearly all cases.
(b)   Subhyaloid haemorrhages occur.
(c)   Cerebrospinal fluid examination may show xanthochromia.
(d)   Leakage or rupture of a berry aneurysm is the commonest aetiology.
(e)   Glycosuria may be found.

9.36

(a)	FALSE	–	Most commoniy presents in the 35–45 year age group.
(b)	FALSE	–	Lower motor neurone palsy.
(c)	TRUE	–	Almost invariably.
(d)	TRUE		
(e)	TRUE	–	Also vertigo.

9.37

(a)	TRUE	–	Particularly if frontal.
(b)	TRUE	–	Hepatic failure also.
(c)	TRUE		
(d)	TRUE	–	As can manganese, lead and alcohol.
(e)	TRUE		

9.38

(a)	TRUE	–	Part of Wernicke's encephalopathy, seen usually in alcoholics nowadays.
(b)	TRUE	–	This is part of Korsakoff's psychosis.
(c)	TRUE		
(d)	TRUE		
(e)	TRUE	–	This may persist despite giving intravenous thiamine treatment. Ocular palsies do tend to resolve with appropriate treatment.

9.39

(a)	TRUE	–	Also vertigo and vomiting, often of abrupt onset.
(b)	FALSE	–	Contralateral loss in the body, ipsilateral in the face.
(c)	TRUE		
(d)	TRUE	–	Due to brain stem involvement.
(e)	TRUE		

9.40

(a)	FALSE	–	Consciousness may or may not be lost.
(b)	TRUE	–	Unilateral or bilateral. Papilloedema can also occur.
(c)	TRUE	–	Uniform blood staining.
(d)	TRUE	–	Other causes include leakage or rupture of angioma or arteriovenous malformation.
(e)	TRUE	–	Also proteinuria in some cases.

9.41 **Characteristic features of a chronic subdural haematoma are:**
(a) Headache.
(b) History of head injury in all cases.
(c) Papilloedema.
(d) Contralateral hemiplegia.
(e) Fluctuating consciousness level.

9.42 **The following can cause seizures:**
(a) Hypoglycaemia.
(b) Hypocalcaemia.
(c) Toxoplasmosis.
(d) Cocaine.
(e) Meningitis.

9.43 **Cord compression is a recognized complication of:**
(a) Paget's disease.
(b) Hodgkin's disease.
(c) Anterior protrusion of a vertebral disc.
(d) Pott's disease.
(e) Neurofibromatosis.

9.44 **Recognized causes of a Charcot joint are:**
(a) Syringomyelia.
(b) Peroneal muscular atrophy.
(c) Diabetes mellitus.
(d) Yaws.
(e) Tabes dorsalis.

9.45 **In the investigation of a patient with meningococcal meningitis, expected findings would include:**
(a) Purpuric rash.
(b) Decreased cerebrospinal fluid (CSF) protein level.
(c) Gram-negative bacilli in the cerebrospinal fluid.
(d) Increased CSF lymphocyte count.
(e) Low CSF glucose concentration.

9.41
(a)	TRUE	– In approximately 75% of cases.
(b)	FALSE	– It often follows a trivial head injury but can occur spontaneously.
(c)	TRUE	– Due to increased intracranial pressure.
(d)	TRUE	
(e)	TRUE	– Other symptoms such as headache may also vary from day to day.

9.42
(a)	TRUE	
(b)	TRUE	– Other metabolic causes are renal or hepatic failure.
(c)	TRUE	– Commonest intracranial lesion in AIDS.
(d)	TRUE	– Also lignocaine, alcohol and barbiturate withdrawal.
(e)	TRUE	– Also encephalitis.

9.43
(a)	TRUE	
(b)	TRUE	
(c)	FALSE	– Posterior protrusion can.
(d)	TRUE	
(e)	TRUE	– 'Dumb bell' tumour.

9.44
(a)	TRUE	– Can cause Charcot joints in the upper limbs.
(b)	FALSE	– Can produce pes cavus.
(c)	TRUE	
(d)	TRUE	– Also syphilis.
(e)	TRUE	

9.45
(a)	TRUE	
(b)	FALSE	– This is increased; also raised in pneumococcal, *H.influenzae* and TB meningitis.
(c)	FALSE	– Gram-negative diplococci.
(d)	FALSE	– Increase in polymorphs.
(e)	TRUE	

9.46 **Causes of a raised CSF protein are:**
(a) Guillain–Barré syndrome.
(b) Acoustic neuroma.
(c) Multiple sclerosis.
(d) Thyrotoxicosis.
(e) Spinal tumour.

9.47 **Recognized associations of neurofibromatosis are:**
(a) Phaeochromocytoma.
(b) Aortic stenosis.
(c) Berry aneurysms.
(d) Pes cavus.
(e) Café au lait spots.

9.48 **Complications of herpes zoster infections include:**
(a) Muscle wasting.
(b) Encephalitis.
(c) Corneal ulceration.
(d) Post-herpetic neuralgia.
(e) Hyperacusis.

9.49 **Extradural haematoma:**
(a) Is more common in females than males.
(b) Is usually associated with a skull fracture.
(c) Usually presents 4–6 weeks after the original injury.
(d) Can be treated conservatively.
(e) Results most commonly from trauma to the basilar artery.

9.50 **Cerebral infarction is associated with:**
(a) Fat embolism.
(b) Hypertension.
(c) Bacterial endocarditis.
(d) Carbon monoxide poisoning.
(e) Polyarteritis nodosa.

9.46

(a)	TRUE	– Can be very high.
(b)	TRUE	
(c)	TRUE	
(d)	FALSE	– Hypothyroidism can.
(e)	TRUE	

9.47

(a)	TRUE	
(b)	FALSE	– Coarctation of the aorta is associated.
(c)	TRUE	
(d)	TRUE	
(e)	TRUE	– Other cutaneous manifestations are fibromas (soft, pink swellings) which can be numerous.

9.48

(a)	TRUE	– Can get segmental muscle wasting due to infection of the motor root.
(b)	TRUE	– In the immunosuppressed.
(c)	TRUE	– In ophthalmic herpes.
(d)	TRUE	– This has an increased incidence in the elderly.
(e)	TRUE	– Due to paralysis of the nerve to stapedius in geniculate herpes zoster.

9.49

(a)	FALSE	– No difference between the sexes.
(b)	TRUE	
(c)	FALSE	– Usually within the first day (usually within a few hours).
(d)	FALSE	– Surgical emergency.
(e)	FALSE	– Due to middle meningeal artery damage.

9.50

(a)	TRUE	– As are other causes of cerebral embolism.
(b)	TRUE	– One of the principal causes.
(c)	TRUE	– Can cause cerebral emboli.
(d)	TRUE	– Causes cerebral hypoxia.
(e)	TRUE	– As can SLE.

9.51 **The following drugs are typically used in the treatment of depression:**
(a) Dexfenfluramine hydrochloride.
(b) Mianserin.
(c) Desipramine.
(d) Paroxetine.
(e) Pizotifen.

9.52 **Parkinsonism is a recognized complication of:**
(a) Haloperidol.
(b) Chlorpropamide.
(c) Methyldopa.
(d) Manganese.
(e) Reserpine.

9.53 **The following typically occur in an overdose of tricyclic antidepressants:**
(a) Respiratory depression.
(b) Bullous lesions.
(c) Pinpoint pupils.
(d) Convulsions.
(e) Arrhythmias.

9.54 **Chorea is associated with:**
(a) L-dopa therapy.
(b) Prednisolone.
(c) Wilson's disease.
(d) Rheumatoid disease.
(e) SLE.

9.55 **Duchenne muscular dystrophy:**
(a) Usually causes death in those affected before 20 years of age.
(b) Is an autosomal recessive condition.
(c) Is associated with intellectual retardation in almost all cases.
(d) May lead to hypertrophy of the calf muscles.
(e) May present with delayed onset of walking.

9.51
(a)   FALSE   –   Appetite suppressant (Adifax).
(b)   TRUE
(c)   TRUE   –   Tricyclic antidepressant.
(d)   TRUE   –   Serotonin reuptake blocker.
(e)   FALSE   –   Used in migraine treatment.

9.52
(a)   TRUE   –   Dystonic movements are more common than in idiopathic Parkinson's disease.
(b)   FALSE   –   Chlorpromazine and other phenothiazines can.
(c)   TRUE
(d)   TRUE   –   Copper can also cause Parkinsonism.
(e)   TRUE

9.53
(a)   TRUE   –   Also hypotension and hypothermia.
(b)   FALSE   –   This is due to barbiturates.
(c)   FALSE   –   Dilated pupils.
(d)   TRUE
(e)   TRUE

9.54
(a)   TRUE
(b)   FALSE   –   Oral contraceptive pill can.
(c)   TRUE   –   Other features are dementia and emotional lability.
(d)   FALSE   –   Sydenham's chorea and Huntington's chorea are rare causes.
(e)   TRUE

9.55
(a)   TRUE   –   Usually from respiratory infection or cardiac failure.
(b)   FALSE   –   It is an X-linked recessive condition.
(c)   FALSE   –   This is found in about 20% of cases.
(d)   TRUE   –   Due to hypertrophy of gastrocnemius and soleus muscles.
(e)   TRUE   –   Other presenting features are falls and an inability to run.

9.56 **Normal pressure hydrocephalus is characterized by:**
(a) Small ventricles on CT scanning.
(b) Dementia.
(c) Apraxia.
(d) Ataxia.
(e) Urinary incontinence.

9.57 **Recognized features of temporal lobe seizures are:**
(a) Disturbance of conscious level.
(b) Déjà-vu phenomenon.
(c) Paresis in the affected limbs for a few days post-epileptic attack.
(d) Hallucinations of smell.
(e) Two to three cycles per second generalized spike and wave pattern on EEG.

9.58 **Cerebral aneurysms are associated with:**
(a) Hypertension.
(b) Polycystic disease of the kidney.
(c) Subacute bacterial endocarditis.
(d) Friedreich's ataxia.
(e) Wegener's granulomatosis.

9.59 **Cataract formation is known to be associated with:**
(a) Diabetes mellitus.
(b) Hyperparathyroidism.
(c) Irradiation.
(d) Myasthenia gravis.
(e) Down's syndrome.

9.60 **Non-metastatic neurological complications of carcinoma include:**
(a) Narcolepsy.
(b) Dementia.
(c) Cerebellar ataxia.
(d) Peripheral neuropathy.
(e) Eaton Lambert syndrome.

9.56

(a)	FALSE	–	Enlarged ventricles on CT. Ventricular shunting can result in improvement.
(b)	TRUE	–	There may be fluctuating confusion.
(c)	TRUE	–	Gait apraxia.
(d)	TRUE	–	Also extensor plantar reflexes.
(e)	TRUE		

9.57

(a)	TRUE	–	Consciousness is altered but not necessarily lost.
(b)	TRUE		
(c)	FALSE	–	This is Todd's paralysis, following focal epilepsy.
(d)	TRUE		
(e)	FALSE	–	Petit mal epilepsy.

9.58

(a)	TRUE		
(b)	TRUE		
(c)	TRUE	–	Causing a mycotic aneurysm.
(d)	FALSE		
(e)	TRUE	–	Also polyarteritis nodosa.

9.59

(a)	TRUE	–	Snowflake cataract (uncommon) or increased incidence of 'senile' cataract.
(b)	FALSE	–	Hypoparathyroidism.
(c)	TRUE		
(d)	FALSE	–	Dystrophia myotonica.
(e)	TRUE		

9.60

(a)	FALSE		
(b)	TRUE		
(c)	TRUE		
(d)	TRUE	–	Can be motor, sensory or mixed.
(e)	TRUE	–	Commonest cause is small cell lung cancer.

10 Dermatology

10.1 The following statements are correct:
(a) Bullae consist of collections of purulent fluid.
(b) Macules are firm, raised lesions.
(c) Lichenification is thickening of the skin with increased skin markings.
(d) Crusts are masses of dead tissue from the epidermis.
(e) Vesicles are small collections of fluid with well-defined borders.

10.2 Recognized causes of leg ulcers include:
(a) Psoriasis.
(b) Rheumatic fever.
(c) Sickle-cell anaemia.
(d) Tabes dorsalis.
(e) Pyoderma gangrenosum.

10.3 The following may cause a diffuse increase in skin pigmentation:
(a) Wilson's disease.
(b) Pellagra.
(c) Systemic sclerosis.
(d) Tuberose sclerosis.
(e) Acromegaly.

10.4 Erythema nodosum is associated with:
(a) Tuberculosis.
(b) Diabetes mellitus.
(c) Crohn's disease.
(d) Oral contraceptive pill.
(e) Streptococcal infection.

10.5 The following drugs are recognized to cause photosensitivity:
(a) Cotrimoxazole.
(b) Chlorpromazine.
(c) Ferrous sulphate.
(d) Cephradine.
(e) Amiodarone.

10.1

(a)   FALSE   –   Pustules consist of purulent fluid. Bullae are large vesicles (see (e)).

(b)   FALSE   –   Macules are flat, circumscribed lesions, not raised above the skin.

(c)   TRUE

(d)   FALSE   –   Crusts are composed of bacteria, leucocytes and exudate.

(e)   TRUE

10.2

(a)   FALSE

(b)   FALSE   –   Rheumatoid arthritis can.

(c)   TRUE

(d)   TRUE   –   Other causes are diabetes mellitus and leprosy.

(e)   TRUE

10.3

(a)   TRUE   –   Other causes are haemochromatosis and primary biliary cirrhosis.

(b)   TRUE

(c)   TRUE   –   Also SLE, dermatomyositis.

(d)   FALSE   –   This produces areas of depigmentation.

(e)   TRUE

10.4

(a)   TRUE   –   Also sarcoidosis.

(b)   FALSE

(c)   TRUE   –   Also ulcerative colitis.

(d)   TRUE   –   Sulphonamides also.

(e)   TRUE   –   Probably the commonest cause.

10.5

(a)   TRUE   –   Due to the sulphonamide component.

(b)   TRUE   –   As can other phenothiazines.

(c)   FALSE

(d)   FALSE

(e)   TRUE

10.6 **Pruritus is a recognized complication of:**
(a) Breast carcinoma.
(b) Myxoedema.
(c) Iron deficiency anaemia.
(d) Chronic renal failure.
(e) Phenytoin therapy.

10.7 **Dermatitis herpetiformis:**
(a) Is characterised by a petechial rash.
(b) Is associated with HLA B8.
(c) Mainly affects the mouth.
(d) Is associated with ulcerative colitis.
(e) Usually responds to dapsone treatment.

10.8 **Mucosal ulceration is typical of the following conditions:**
(a) Herpes zoster.
(b) Pernicious anaemia.
(c) Behçet's disease.
(d) Stevens–Johnson syndrome.
(e) Eczema.

10.9 **The following conditions are associated with each other:**
(a) Palmar erythema and cirrhosis.
(b) Lupus pernio and sarcoidosis.
(c) Café au lait spots and porphyria.
(d) Acanthosis nigricans and lung carcinoma.
(e) Necrobiosis lipoidica and thyrotoxicosis.

10.10 **Characteristic features of Behçet's disease include:**
(a) Neutropenia.
(b) Genital ulceration.
(c) Retinitis pigmentosa.
(d) Arthralgia.
(e) Haemoptysis.

10.6
(a)	TRUE	–	As can other carcinomas, e.g. lung, colon.
(b)	TRUE	–	Thyrotoxicosis can also.
(c)	TRUE	–	Other haematological causes include myeloproliferative disorders.
(d)	TRUE		
(e)	FALSE		

10.7
(a)	FALSE	–	Usually macules and papules, then vesicles and bullae.
(b)	TRUE	–	In approximately 80% of cases.
(c)	FALSE	–	Usually affects elbows, knees, scapular and gluteal regions.
(d)	FALSE	–	Associated with a gluten-sensitive enteropathy (may be subclinical).
(e)	TRUE		

10.8
(a)	FALSE		
(b)	FALSE	–	Agranulocytic ulcers occur in aplastic anaemia.
(c)	TRUE		
(d)	TRUE		
(e)	FALSE	–	No mouth involvement.

10.9
(a)	TRUE		
(b)	TRUE		
(c)	FALSE	–	Café au lait spots are found with neurofibromatosis.
(d)	TRUE		
(e)	FALSE	–	Necrobiosis lipoidica is associated with diabetes mellitus.

10.10
(a)	FALSE	–	Raised ESR and neutrophilia.
(b)	TRUE	–	Also oral ulceration.
(c)	FALSE	–	Iritis.
(d)	TRUE		
(e)	TRUE	–	Other features are thrombophlebitis and erythema nodosum.

10.11 Palmar hyperkeratosis is a recognized finding in:
(a) Pseudopolyposis coli.
(b) Osteoporosis.
(c) Anaemia.
(d) Pregnancy.
(e) Psoriasis.

10.12 Pemphigus vulgaris is characterized by:
(a) Subepidermal bullae.
(b) Lesions in the mouth.
(c) Autosomal recessive mode of inheritance.
(d) Absent Nicolsky's sign.
(e) Onset usually in the over 70s.

10.13 Recognized causes of purpura include:
(a) Meningococcal meningitis.
(b) Lichen planus.
(c) Scurvy.
(d) Leukaemia.
(e) Chloramphenicol.

10.14 Cutaneous manifestations of internal malignancy include:
(a) Hypertrichosis.
(b) Lupus vulgaris.
(c) Herpes zoster.
(d) Tendon xanthomata.
(e) Migratory thrombophlebitis.

10.15 The following would suggest that a pigmented lesion had become malignant:
(a) Decrease in size.
(b) Irregular edge.
(c) Bleeding.
(d) Itching.
(e) Uneven pigmentation.

10.11
(a)	FALSE
(b)	FALSE
(c)	FALSE
(d)	FALSE
(e)	TRUE

10.12
(a)	FALSE	– Intra-epidermal bullae.
(b)	TRUE	– These are sometimes the only evidence of the disease.
(c)	FALSE	
(d)	FALSE	– Nikolsky's sign present; superficial skin layer can be moved over the deeper layer.
(e)	FALSE	– Onset in 40–60s.

10.13
(a)	TRUE	
(b)	FALSE	
(c)	TRUE	– Often found on the thighs.
(d)	TRUE	
(e)	TRUE	– Other causes are sulphonamides, methotrexate and indomethacin.

10.14
(a)	TRUE	– This is excessive hair growth and may occur in cachexia.
(b)	FALSE	– Sign of tuberculosis.
(c)	TRUE	– Particularly associated with lymphoma and leukaemia.
(d)	FALSE	
(e)	TRUE	– Especially pancreatic carcinoma.

10.15
(a)	FALSE	– Increase in size would suggest malignancy.
(b)	TRUE	
(c)	TRUE	
(d)	TRUE	
(e)	TRUE	

10.16 Basal cell carcinoma:
(a) Has a rapid onset.
(b) Is the commonest form of skin cancer.
(c) Metastasizes readily early in the course of the disease.
(d) Characteristically has a raised, pearly edge.
(e) Occurs most often on the scalp.

10.17 Characteristic features of pityriasis rosea are:
(a) Scaling of the lesion.
(b) Predominance of lesions on the feet and hands.
(c) Pustular rash.
(d) 'Herald patch'.
(e) Mortality in 5–10% of patients within 2 years.

10.18 Local side-effects of the long-term use of topical corticosteroids include:
(a) Basal cell carcinoma.
(b) Increased hair growth.
(c) Purpura.
(d) Thickening of the dermis.
(e) Acne.

10.19 Psoriasis:
(a) Occurs 10 times as commonly in men than women.
(b) Is predominantly a disease of the elderly.
(c) Is characterized by a purpuric rash.
(d) Affects 1 in 10 000 people in the UK.
(e) Predisposes to squamous cell carcinoma of the skin.

10.20 Characteristic features of psoriasis include:
(a) Scaly rash.
(b) Involvement of the extensor surfaces of limbs.
(c) Nail pitting.
(d) Iritis.
(e) Mononeuritis multiplex.

10.16
(a) FALSE – Insidious onset.
(b) TRUE
(c) FALSE – They rarely metastasize but can cause local ulceration.
(d) TRUE
(e) FALSE – Most common on face and forehead.

10.17
(a) TRUE – Early on the scaling is central, later the scaling is at the edges of the lesion.
(b) FALSE – Most common on trunk and proximal part of limbs.
(c) FALSE – Macular or maculopapular.
(d) TRUE – This is a solitary lesion which precedes rash by 7–10 days.
(e) FALSE – Benign condition.

10.18
(a) FALSE
(b) TRUE
(c) TRUE – Also skin atrophy.
(d) FALSE
(e) TRUE

10.19
(a) FALSE – Equal sex incidence.
(b) FALSE – Most commonly affects those aged 15–30 years, although can affect any age.
(c) FALSE – Papular rash or plaques.
(d) FALSE – Affects 1–2% of the population.
(e) FALSE

10.20
(a) TRUE – Thickness of the scale varies.
(b) TRUE – But any area of skin can be affected, e.g. scalp, back.
(c) TRUE – Also arthropathy in 5–10%.
(d) FALSE
(e) FALSE

10.21 The following are recognized treatments for ps
(a) Griseofulvin.
(b) Dithranol.
(c) Oral steroids.
(d) Methotrexate.
(e) Psoralens and ultraviolet A.

10.22 The following diseases are caused by yeasts:
(a) Candidiasis.
(b) Pityriasis rosea.
(c) Lichen planus.
(d) Tinea capitis.
(e) Pityriasis versicolor.

10.23 Candidiasis:
(a) Is associated with the use of inhaled steroids.
(b) Causes paronychia.
(c) May lead to an abnormal barium swallow.
(d) Causes glossitis.
(e) Occurs more commonly in people with hypothyroidism than in the general population.

10.24 Warts:
(a) Do not remit spontaneously.
(b) Are caused by viruses of the Papova group.
(c) Are best treated by surgical excision.
(d) Undergo malignant change in 10% of cases.
(e) Are only spread by direct contact.

10.25 Chickenpox:
(a) Can cause pulmonary calcification.
(b) Has an incubation period of 4–7 days.
(c) Is treated by tetracycline.
(d) Is caused by the varicella-zoster virus.
(e) Characteristically affects the limbs.

10.21
(a)	FALSE	– This is an antifungal agent.
(b)	TRUE	
(c)	FALSE	
(d)	TRUE	– Folate antagonist.
(e)	TRUE	– 'PUVA'. Psoralen tablets are taken 2 h prior to UVA light exposure.

10.22
(a)	TRUE	– 'Thrush'.
(b)	FALSE	– May be caused by a virus.
(c)	FALSE	– Cause of this is unknown.
(d)	FALSE	– Scalp ringworm.
(e)	TRUE	– Yeast infection with *Pityrosporum orbiculare*.

10.23
(a)	TRUE	– Leading to intra-oral thrush.
(b)	FALSE	– *Candida* infection is secondary.
(c)	TRUE	– Barium is seen to adhere to the areas of candidiasis.
(d)	TRUE	
(e)	FALSE	– More common in diabetes mellitus, alcoholics, AIDS, leukaemia, etc.

10.24
(a)	FALSE	– They do: approximately 10–20% within 3 months.
(b)	TRUE	– Genus papillomavirus.
(c)	FALSE	– Many do not need treatment. Topical wart paints are often used or cryotherapy with liquid nitrogen.
(d)	FALSE	– Malignant change has been reported rarely in Condylomata acuminata.
(e)	FALSE	– Can be spread, e.g. by towels.

10.25
(a)	TRUE	– In adults; it may be permanent.
(b)	FALSE	– Incubation period 12–21 days.
(c)	FALSE	– Treatment is usually symptomatic. If superimposed skin infection, flucloxacillin may be indicated.
(d)	TRUE	
(e)	FALSE	– Mainly affects the trunk and face.

10.26 Causes of scarring alopecia include:
(a) Acromegaly.
(b) Anticoagulants.
(c) Lichen planus.
(d) Iron deficiency anaemia.
(e) Thyrotoxicosis.

10.27 The following characteristically produce 'bullous' lesions:
(a) Trichotillomania.
(b) Seborrhoeic dermatitis.
(c) Epidermolysis bullosa.
(d) Erythema multiforme.
(e) Pemphigoid.

10.28 Paget's disease of the nipple:
(a) Has an acute onset.
(b) Occurs exclusively in females.
(c) Is almost always bilateral.
(d) May resemble eczema.
(e) Is best treated with topical steroids.

10.29 Solar keratosis:
(a) Occurs most commonly on sun-exposed areas of the body.
(b) Is most common in dark-skinned people.
(c) Can undergo malignant change.
(d) Is characterized by brownish hyperkeratotic lesions.
(e) Is usually painful to touch.

10.30 Terbinafine:
(a) May be applied topically.
(b) Is used in the treatment of long-standing *Tinea pedis*.
(c) Decreases the metabolism of warfarin.
(d) Is safe in renal disease.
(e) Is usually given for a maximum course of 7 days.

10.26
(a)   FALSE   –   This can cause hirsutism.
(b)   FALSE   –   Cytotoxics, the oral contraceptive pill and anticoagulants can cause non-scarring alopecia.
(c)   TRUE
(d)   FALSE
(e)   FALSE   –   Hypothyroidism, and rarely thyrotoxicosis, can cause non-scarring alopecia.

10.27
(a)   FALSE   –   Disorder where the individual pulls out their own hair.
(b)   FALSE
(c)   TRUE   –   Congenital disorder.
(d)   TRUE
(e)   TRUE   –   Also pemphigus.

10.28
(a)   FALSE   –   Chronic onset.
(b)   FALSE   –   Can rarely affect males.
(c)   FALSE   –   Unilateral.
(d)   TRUE   –   This is usually bilateral and responds to simple measures.
(e)   FALSE   –   Requires surgical intervention, as well as radiotherapy in some cases.

10.29
(a)   TRUE   –   For instance on the scalp and face.
(b)   FALSE   –   More common in fair-skinned people.
(c)   TRUE   –   Although this is not common.
(d)   TRUE
(e)   FALSE

10.30
(a)   TRUE   –   Also available orally.
(b)   TRUE
(c)   FALSE   –   No effect on warfarin metabolism.
(d)   FALSE
(e)   FALSE   –   It may be needed for 2–6 weeks in *Tinea pedis*, or even longer, e.g. *Tinea capitis*.

10.31 Adult atopic eczema:
(a) Is always preceded by a history of childhood eczema.
(b) Is worsened by local steroid application.
(c) Only affects the extensor aspects of the limbs.
(d) Is associated with a family history of atopy.
(e) Causes pruritus.

10.32 Hirsutism is associated with:
(a) Pregnancy.
(b) Diabetes mellitus.
(c) Cushing's syndrome.
(d) Hypothyroidism.
(e) Anabolic steroids.

10.33 Recognized manifestations of SLE include:
(a) Sclerodactyly.
(b) Alopecia.
(c) Photosensitivity.
(d) Nasal ulceration.
(e) Persistent urticaria.

10.34 Characteristic features of dermatomyositis include:
(a) Cataracts.
(b) Nailfold infarcts.
(c) Purple discolouration around the eyes.
(d) Skin ulcers.
(e) Telangiectasia.

10.35 Recognized causes of erythema multiforme include:
(a) Sulphonamides.
(b) Herpes simplex infection.
(c) Mycoplasma infection.
(d) Phenytoin.
(e) Sulphonylureas.

10.31
(a)	FALSE	– There may not be such a history.
(b)	FALSE	– This is often beneficial.
(c)	FALSE	– Flexures, face and neck are commonly affected.
(d)	TRUE	
(e)	TRUE	– Can be severe.

10.32
(a)	TRUE	
(b)	FALSE	
(c)	TRUE	– As can exogenous steroids.
(d)	FALSE	
(e)	TRUE	– Also adrenal tumours and congenital adrenal hyperplasia.

10.33
(a)	FALSE	– This is found in systemic sclerosis.
(b)	TRUE	
(c)	TRUE	
(d)	TRUE	– Also buccal ulceration.
(e)	TRUE	

10.34
(a)	FALSE	
(b)	TRUE	
(c)	TRUE	– 'Heliotrope' colour.
(d)	FALSE	– This is typical of scleroderma.
(e)	TRUE	– Can involve face, trunk, arms.

10.35
(a)	TRUE	– Other drug causes are barbiturates, penicillin and salicylates.
(b)	TRUE	– As can glandular or rheumatic fever.
(c)	TRUE	
(d)	TRUE	
(e)	TRUE	

10.36 Stevens–Johnson syndrome:
(a) May be complicated by pneumonia.
(b) Can cause visual damage.
(c) Does not involve the buccal cavity.
(d) Is characteristically associated with target lesions.
(e) Usually remits in 6–8 weeks.

10.37 Scabies:
(a) Is caused by *Pediculosis corporis*.
(b) Is transmitted by close contact.
(c) Typically causes itching worse at night.
(d) Characteristically burrows in the web spaces of the fingers.
(e) Is treated with benzoyl peroxide.

10.38 Recognized findings in Reiter's disease include:
(a) Mouth ulcers.
(b) Conjunctivitis.
(c) Circinate balanitis.
(d) Keratoderma blenorrhagica.
(e) Nail thickening.

10.39 Erythroderma:
(a) Occurs predominantly in children.
(b) Does not cause pruritus.
(c) Can complicate eczema.
(d) Produces a pustular rash.
(e) Is associated with lymphadenopathy.

10.40 Rosacea:
(a) Is a papular pustular rash.
(b) Commonly involves the central area of the face.
(c) Can be aggravated by excessive alcohol intake.
(d) Is best treated with topical corticosteroids.
(e) Is more common in men than women.

10.36

(a)	TRUE		
(b)	TRUE	–	Due to keratitis or conjunctival scarring.
(c)	FALSE	–	May cause mucosal ulceration.
(d)	TRUE	–	Rings of erythema of differing intensities.
(e)	TRUE	–	May need treatment with oral steroids.

10.37

(a)	FALSE	–	Caused by *Sarcoptes scabiei* (*Acarus scabiei*).
(b)	TRUE		
(c)	TRUE	–	When the person is warm.
(d)	TRUE	–	Also flexor surface of wrists, palms, areolae of nipples.
(e)	FALSE	–	Treated with permethrin. Older treatments include benzyl benzoate.

10.38

(a)	TRUE		
(b)	TRUE	–	Iritis in chronic disease.
(c)	TRUE	–	Skin ulceration of the glans and prepuce.
(d)	TRUE	–	Pustular hyperkeratotic lesions on the soles, sometimes on the palms.
(e)	TRUE		

10.39

(a)	FALSE	–	Most common in middle age.
(b)	FALSE	–	Can be severe itching.
(c)	TRUE	–	Can complicate other skin disorders, e.g. psoriasis, seborrhoeic dermatitis.
(d)	FALSE	–	Macular rash, which coalesces. Skin can become generally red.
(e)	TRUE		

10.40

(a)	TRUE	–	Also redness but no comedones.
(b)	TRUE	–	May be more widespread than this.
(c)	TRUE		
(d)	FALSE	–	Topically, e.g. metronidazole. Tetracyclines orally are beneficial.
(e)	FALSE	–	Women predominate.